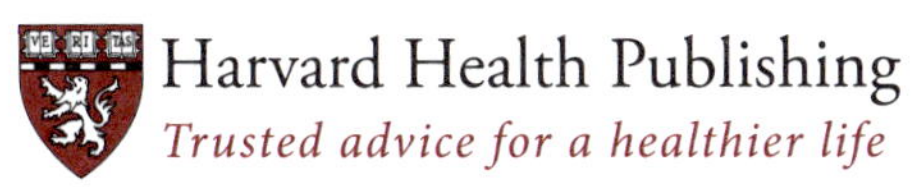

Dear Reader,

Balance is a complex phenomenon, involving your eyes, ears, muscles, and brain. It's something you may take for granted … until you suffer a serious fall. When toddlers tumble, they may shed a few tears before surging ahead again unscathed. But when an adult falls, particularly an older adult, consequences are often far worse, potentially leading to a hip fracture, head injury, or even death.

In young, healthy adults, balance is largely an automatic reflex. As you move into your 50s and 60s, however, you may notice yourself becoming less stable. Gradual changes linked to growing older—such as loss of muscle mass, slower reflexes, and worsening eyesight—can affect your sense of balance. Certain health problems—such as inner ear disorders, hearing loss, heart rhythm disturbances, and neuropathy (nerve damage that causes weakness, numbness, and pain)—may upset balance, too. So can the use of alcohol and certain medications.

Shaky balance can lead to a downward spiral. Often, you begin moving around less during the day, voluntarily cutting back on activities. Then confidence dips, muscles essential to balance grow weaker, and unsteadiness increases in response. So does the fear of falling—which in turn may further constrain your activities.

There's a real "use it or lose it" component to balance. Whether you're looking to prevent balance issues or reverse them, you need to challenge your balance on a regular basis. That's why we've combined our expertise to bring you a range of safe, effective exercises that can improve your balance, flexibility, and strength. As you'll see, some of the workouts are easier and some are harder, to accommodate people with varying degrees of balance issues. But with practice, almost anyone—of any age—can achieve better balance. What's more, the full blend of recommended activities can help you build better awareness of your body and surroundings, boost your confidence, and tune up your heart and lungs to keep you healthy and independent.

Falls occur for many reasons, of course—not just balance problems. Clutter, broken pavement, dim lighting, and even essential medications can play a role. Our checklists offer step-by-step strategies for fall-proofing yourself and your home. So, read the safety and fall-prevention tips. Talk to your doctor about any health problems and medications that might increase your risk for falls. Then get started on the exercises. Fewer injuries, restored confidence, and a renewed zest for life are well worth the effort.

Sincerely,

Suzanne Salamon, M.D. *Medical Editor*	Brad Manor, Ph.D. *Medical Editor*	Michele Stanten *Fitness Consultant*

How balance works

To watch a tightrope walker slink across a wire high above the ground is to appreciate what a finely honed sense of balance can do. But everyday tasks, too, require more complex coordination than you may realize. Just observe a baby's tentative first steps as he or she tries to find a center of balance, hold the body upright, and transfer weight successfully from one foot to the other even once or twice. Then the truth hits home. It is no simple thing that we two-legged humans do day in, day out, for most of our lives.

It takes many parts of the body, working together flawlessly and with great precision, to achieve a good sense of balance. But beginning in your 50s, you may start noticing subtle changes. Perhaps you don't feel quite as secure perching on a ladder, or maybe you find that you're paying closer attention to your footing when going down stairs. These things are unlikely to slow you down much at this stage. But during your workouts, it may be useful to challenge yourself from time to time with balance exercises.

As time moves on, you may find that poor balance becomes a more serious problem. For older adults in particular, balance is essential to maintaining good health, since physical activity becomes difficult without it. Poor balance not only restricts your movements, but it can also lead to falls and resulting injuries. And in the elderly, one fall can lead to fear of another fall, which further restricts activity.

Good balance, by contrast, helps prevent falls. It builds confidence and fosters independence. If you are still active, it can help improve your tennis, golf, running, dancing, skating, skiing, or any number of other sports or activities. Not an athlete? Simple actions like climbing in and out of the bathtub, going up and down stairs, picking up a child or grandchild, and even turning to look behind you require good balance, too.

Fortunately, there are many ways to help improve your balance. The next chapter addresses some of the medical and age-related issues that contribute to poor balance. Though some of them cannot be fixed, others have remedies you may be able to tackle with your doctor, such as keeping blood pressure from falling too low or making sure you have the right prescription in your glasses. The Special Section (see page 13) also includes checklists of action items for personal health and home safety that can help prevent falls.

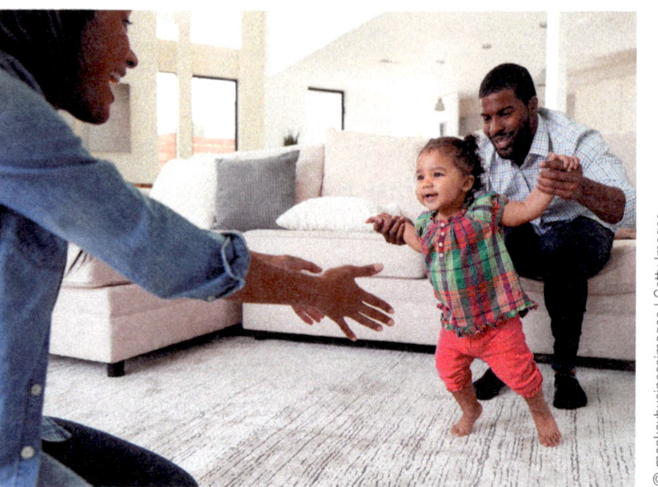

A baby's first tentative steps show just how complicated balance is. It takes many parts of the body, working together flawlessly and with great precision, to achieve a good sense of balance.

Once you have dealt with any issues that may be causing balance problems or fall risks, the most important thing you can do is to start practicing balance exercises. These exercises can hone your balance in multiple ways. For example, they work together to

- sharpen your reflexive responses
- improve your brain's ability to integrate sensory feedback and make split-second calls on how to correct any imbalances
- strengthen and coordinate commands from your brain to your muscles
- tone your muscles, so they are better able to respond to commands from the brain
- improve your posture and strengthen your core, so you can maintain a more stable stance.

By doing all this and more, the exercises in this

The trouble with falls

- Falls are the leading cause of accidental death in older adults. Every 15 minutes, an older adult dies from a fall-related injury.
- Every 11 seconds, an adult age 65 or older is treated in the emergency department for an injury from a fall.
- One out of five falls leads to a fracture (broken bone), a blow to the head, or another serious problem.
- Nearly half of hospitalizations for traumatic brain injuries are the result of falls.
- Roughly 80% of all falls occur in the home. The most common sites are bedrooms, bathrooms, and stairs.
- Men are more likely than women to fall outdoors and to die from falls.
- Women are more likely to fall indoors and be injured.
- Older women have more than twice the rate of fall-related fractures compared with men, perhaps because they are more likely to suffer from osteoporosis.
- Practically all hip fractures—over 95%—result from falls. Over 300,000 older adults are hospitalized each year because of hip fractures.
- Complications following a hip fracture or surgery to treat it, such as pneumonia or blood clots, are sometimes fatal.
- The biggest risk factor for future falls is having had a previous fall.

report will help make you steadier, more confident, and less likely to fall. We've designed progressive challenges, starting with three safe, easy balance workouts that should be within reach for people of all ages. Because some of our readers are younger and looking to head off future trouble, we've also included three harder routines that provide greater challenges. Practicing any of these routines regularly will help prevent declines in your balance—and may noticeably improve it.

In addition, after completing any of the balance workouts, we suggest a stretching routine to bolster your flexibility. Flexibility can also help prevent falls by improving your agility and range of motion.

Before launching into the exercises, though, it helps to understand how your sense of balance works and how aging, health issues, and various medicines affect it.

The body's balance systems

Balance can be described as the ability to distribute your weight in a way that enables you to hold a steady position or move at will without falling. Static balance helps you stay upright when standing still. Dynamic balance allows you to anticipate and react to changes as you move. Both types of balance work to keep your center of gravity—the point at which body weight is evenly distributed—poised over your base of support.

Whether you're moving or standing still, balance requires interplay among several systems: the central nervous system (brain and spinal cord), the vestibular system (brain and inner ear), the visual system (brain and eyes), and a vast web of position-sensing nerves called proprioceptors in peripheral areas of the body, such as the legs. Muscles and bones are pressed into service as well, to turn spinal reflexes and the brain's commands into movements.

Brain. Together, the brain and spinal cord form the central nervous system. The cerebellum, a portion of the brain perched above the brainstem, helps coordinate balance and movement. It receives information gathered by a network of sensory nerves and issues commands. It also retrieves stored memories of movements deeply ingrained through practice—for example, walking, riding a bike, or kicking a soccer ball. The cerebrum (the largest part of the brain) chimes in, too. Home to the frontal lobe, which plays roles in attention, planning, and movement, this part of the brain helps surmount challenges like a slippery sidewalk or a rocky path.

Spinal cord. Housed safely in a channel carved through the vertebrae, the spinal cord serves as a bridge between the brain and the body. Paired nerves peppered along its length receive feedback from the peripheral nervous system, a lacework of nerve fibers branching out from the central nervous system to the body's extremities. The spinal cord also gives rise to a host of reflexes, such as the quick-stepping response to an unexpected push. It delivers voluntary movement commands to the muscles, too.

Vestibular system. Central to the sense of balance is the vestibular system of the inner ear. It contains several important structures, including three fluid-filled loops called the semicircular canals, which tell your brain the position of your head. At the base of each loop, a bell-shaped structure called a cupula sits above a clump of hairlike sensory cells known as hair cells. As thick fluid (endolymph) in each semicircular canal moves, its cupula tilts, bending the hair cells. Signals set off by this action travel to the brain via the acoustic nerve and describe the position and rotational movements of your head—straight up and down, side to side, tilting toward one shoulder, and so forth.

Two additional sensory organs called the utricle and the saccule are also lined with hair cells, which tell the brain when you're sitting up, leaning back, or lying down. Inside the utricle and saccule, grains of calcium carbonate (called canaliths or otoconia) are sprinkled on top of a layer of gel overlying the hair cells. Each time your head tilts, gravity pulls on these tiny stones. Hair cells shift in response, sending signals to the brain describing the position of your head. The sensory cells in the utricle also report forward motion—say, when you're walking forward or riding a bike. Those in the saccule monitor vertical acceleration of the body, which would occur if you stood up or rode in an elevator, for example.

These five organs in each inner ear provide the brain with enough information on the position and motion of your head that it can maintain your balance the vast majority of the time. However, if you spin around very fast, the fluid in the utricle and saccule can't move fast enough to tell your brain your exact position, so you feel dizzy.

Visual system. The eyes send visual information via the optic nerve to the brain, constantly logging where you are in relation to surrounding objects. Thus, sight is a key supplement to other sensory input and is important to balance. If you doubt this, stand next to a counter and lift one of your feet. Now try closing your eyes while lifting your foot. Odds are good that you'll sway more and need to grab on to the counter to steady yourself.

Proprioceptors. These position-sensing nerves are responsible for proprioception, the ability to perceive where your body is in space. Proprioception helps you stay balanced and move through your environment without stumbling or bumping into things. Found primarily in muscles, tendons, and joints, proprioceptors constantly stream information to the brain. The brain then relays commands back down the chain, instructing muscles to adjust contractions in large or small ways as conditions change—when, for example, you stand on an unsteady surface or step off a curb into the street. Proprioceptors in your feet play an especially big role in balance. As you shift from standing to walking forward, for example, pressure rolls toward the front portion of your foot, an act captured by proprioceptors threaded along the sole of the foot and throughout the ankle joint.

Muscles, tendons, and bones. Strong cords of connective tissue called tendons tether muscles to bones. Sensory information gathered by proprioceptors is transmitted to the brain via lightning-quick signals sent along nerve pathways. Commands from the brain are returned just as speedily, and prompt opposing muscles to contract and release. The muscles attached to tendons tug on bones, causing your body to move as instructed.

Balance problems

A third of Americans, at some point in their lives, will have a balance problem that is disturbing enough that they consult a doctor about it, according to the National Institutes of Health. Changes tied to growing older or health issues may underpin these problems. Medications can cause drowsiness, dizziness, or nerve damage. Tight, inflexible, or weak muscles and poor posture impinge on balance, too. Frequently, a combination of problems is at play. This chapter contains more detailed information about these issues and others.

Investigating balance problems

If you frequently feel unsteady on your feet or suffer from dizziness or vertigo (the sensation of the room spinning), talk with your doctor. Too often balance problems and risks of falling aren't discussed until a condition becomes serious. By identifying and addressing issues early, your doctor can help you avoid future problems.

The process of diagnosing may begin with a physical exam and medication review, plus further testing as needed.

Physical exam

A thorough physical exam can uncover underlying health problems. This is the time to report bothersome symptoms, such as dizziness, vertigo, blurred vision, decreased hearing, or confusion. Sometimes people with balance disorders experience other symptoms, too: nausea and vomiting, heart rate and blood pressure changes, and anxiety or panic. It's important to explain to your doctor when symptoms occur, and whether they are long-lasting or come and go. Any recent illnesses or injuries, particularly from falls, may provide clues, too. For example, even a bad cold can temporarily upset the vestibular system.

Your doctor may take your blood pressure while you're seated, then again immediately after you stand, and possibly a few minutes later. A sudden drop in blood pressure when you change position like this—called orthostatic hypotension—can make you dizzy and increase your risk of falling (see "Blood pressure," page 7).

Your doctor may also check your reflexes and range of motion (how far you can move a joint in a given direction), particularly in your lower body. Report any joint stiffness or soreness, as these may limit your agility and balance. You may be asked to do a few basic balance tests under supervision. A "get up and go test" requires you to rise from a chair without pushing off with your arms, and then walk several steps back and forth. This allows your doctor to assess your balance and gait (the speed and rhythm of the way you walk). Taking a few steps with your eyes closed shows whether proprioception is impaired. A basic test of vertigo may be done by moving your head through different positions, which can provide clues about inner ear problems. Tests for peripheral neuropathy (nerve damage that is a long-term complication of diabetes and other conditions), such as the ability to perceive a light touch or vibration on the feet and ankles, may also be done.

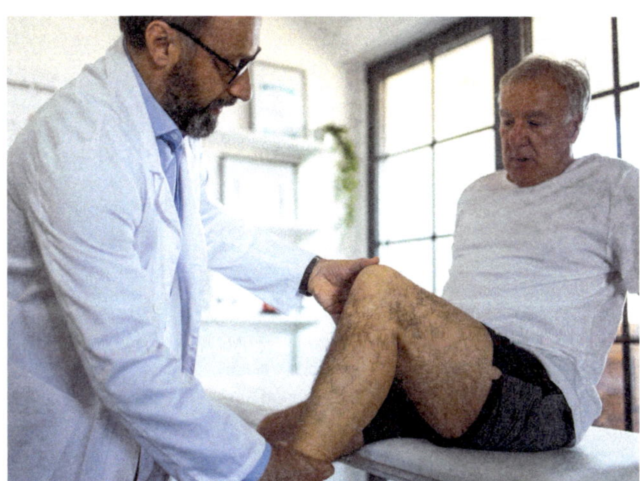

A physical exam can uncover underlying health problems that contribute to poor balance. Your doctor may also check your reflexes and range of motion, particularly in your lower body.

Further tests

Depending on what your doctor learns, further evaluation may require a visit to a specialist, such as an otolaryngologist (an ear, nose, and throat specialist, or ENT) or an otologist (a medical doctor who has additional training in hearing and balance disorders). Further testing varies, but may include any of the following, listed from the most to the least likely to help:

An eye exam will reveal eye disorders like cataracts, glaucoma, diabetic retinopathy, and age-related macular degeneration, which can impair vision. Your eyes play a key role in balance by sending information to your brain about your surroundings. These types of eye disorders can cause blurry vision or spots and floaters that can obstruct your field of vision, leading to falls. Treating these conditions can preserve your eyesight, keep you more sure-footed, and reduce your risk of falling.

A hearing exam could help point to the underlying problem, since hearing and balance are closely connected in the inner ear, and hearing loss has been linked to a higher risk of falling. Several relevant tests may be done, according to the Vestibular Disorders Association. For example, an otoacoustic emissions test assesses the responsiveness of the hair cells lining the cochlea (a spiral-shaped organ in the inner ear that is essential to hearing), and an auditory brainstem response test tracks nerve signals from the ear to the brain and within different portions of the brain.

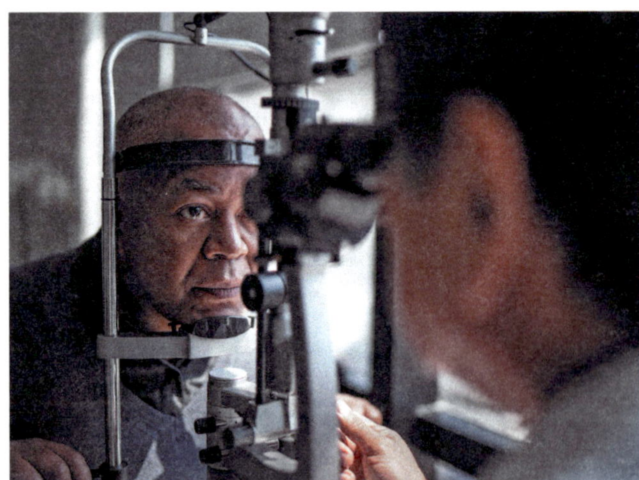

Your eyes play a key role in balance by helping to orient your body. Regular eye exams can pinpoint problems that might impair your vision, and can make sure your eyeglass prescription is up-to-date.

An electrocardiogram (ECG) evaluates your heart's electrical activity. Irregularities may indicate an arrhythmia, which can cause dizziness and falls, or a problem called syncope, in which blood flow to the brain temporarily slows, which can induce fainting.

An echocardiogram will determine if heart valves are functioning properly.

Imaging studies, such as CT or MRI scans of the head and brain, would show any growths or other abnormalities.

A computerized dynamic posturography test employs a movable platform that you stand on. Sensory and motor responses are measured as the platform moves or as visual patterns change.

Videonystagmography uses goggles fitted with infrared cameras to measure eye movements as your head position changes. An older test called electronystagmography uses electrodes to measure muscle movement around the eyes. A rotational chair may be used with either technique.

A caloric reflex test relies on warm or cold water that's squirted into the ear canal to stimulate the acoustic nerve and balance sensors in the inner ear. (The word "caloric" here refers to a unit of heat, not food.) Normally this triggers rapid, side-to-side eye movements called nystagmus. The direction of these movements should vary: the eyes should look first toward and then away from the warm water, and away from and then toward the cold water. The response to testing in both ears should be similar. Often, this test is done during videonystagmography or electronystagmography.

Age-related balance problems

A number of changes ascribed to aging get a surprisingly early start: muscle strength begins dwindling in the 30s, for example, and vision starts declining in the 40s. While you can't sidestep every age-related problem outlined here, you may be able to slow the rate at which some occur, or learn to compensate for changes you can't control. Simply becoming more aware of certain problems may help you stay on your feet, too.

Blood pressure. As you age, your blood pressure tends to rise, increasing your risk for heart attacks and strokes. However, blood pressure that dips suddenly when you stand up is also a problem, particularly for balance, because it causes dizziness, blurry vision, and sometimes fainting. Called orthostatic hypotension or postural hypotension, this problem affects as many as one in three elderly people. Possible causes include dehydration, prolonged bed rest, atherosclerosis (the buildup of fatty deposits in arteries), diabetes, and use of certain medications to treat high blood pressure. Treatment varies, depending on the cause. Standing up slowly—sitting first on the side of the bed when you rise, for example—may help. Consuming adequate liquids is also important. If medications are the problem (see "Medications that affect balance," page 11), talk with your doctor about whether you still need all the drugs you're taking or whether you could substitute another drug for one that's causing problems.

Hearing and vestibular system. Hearing loss often results from damage to hair cells in the cochlea, the snail-shaped auditory organ of the inner ear. Age and cumulative exposure to loud noise gradually harm these cells. Some cells die, leaving fewer to respond to sounds. Similarly, hair cells in the vestibular system deteriorate and die off over time, which may affect accurate detection of head position and movement. Hearing aids may help some people with hearing loss to regain their balance. In the future, hair cell transplants may be another option.

Sight. Visual acuity (the ability to focus and see things clearly) diminishes with age. So do depth perception, night vision, and sensitivity to contrast. When you lose visual cues that help inform you about your surroundings, which direction you're traveling in, and how quickly you're moving, it compromises balance, forcing you to rely more on other senses. Depending on the problem, corrective lenses or surgery such as cataract surgery may be necessary. Brighter, nonglare lighting may help, too.

Muscle strength and power. The average 30-year-old can expect to lose 25% of muscle mass and strength by age 70, plus another 25% by age 90. Weaker muscles aren't the whole story, though. A loss of power—which is a function of both strength and speed—affects balance, too. Faced with a four-lane intersection, you may have the muscle strength to cross the street. But do you have the muscle power needed to do so before the light turns red? At any age, appropriate exercise can help you rebuild strength and power, or at least slow the decline. In many cases, you can take a strength exercise and simply perform it at a faster tempo to turn it into a power exercise. (For a demonstration, watch the video at www.health.harvard.edu/strength-to-power.)

Reflexes. The swift, involuntary protective responses known as reflexes tend to slow with age. Thus, it may take more time to react when you start to stumble or if a pet or child scampers underfoot. People also tend to lose some coordination as they grow older. Damage to nerve pathways or disuse due to a sedentary lifestyle can contribute to the problem. Such changes are another important reason to work on developing muscle strength and power.

Proprioception. Knowing where your body is in relation to its surroundings keeps you from stumbling or bumping up against objects. Proprioception may diminish with age, possibly because of peripheral neuropathy or damage to cells in the inner ear. A cane might help you sense the ground better. Another possibility is a vestibular rehabilitation program consisting of customized exercises designed to improve proprioception. (For help finding a vestibular specialist, contact the Vestibular Disorders Association; see "Resources," page 51.)

Bones. While bone strength rarely affects balance, it can surely affect the aftermath of a fall. As you grow older, your bones become thinner and more fragile. This can lead to low bone mass or osteoporosis, which makes bones much more susceptible to breaking. Low calcium and vitamin D intake, hormonal shifts at menopause, a sedentary lifestyle, smoking, too much alcohol, and long-term use of certain medications can accelerate bone loss.

Health conditions that affect balance

A lengthy list of health problems can interfere with balance. This section briefly outlines some of the more common conditions. Many balance problems, such as those caused by arthritis or milder forms of the eye disorders described below, will respond well to the exercises in the workouts. The exercises can also help counteract mild balance impairments due to stroke, Parkinson's disease, and multiple sclerosis. More severe balance problems that are caused by those conditions are beyond the scope of this report.

To help determine whether you should see a doctor before trying these exercises, see "Starting balance workouts safely," page 20. No matter which underlying problems affect your balance, remember that you can do much to prevent falls by identifying hazards and fixing them, as explained in the checklists. Harvard also has a number of Special Health Reports—including *Coping with Hearing Loss*, *The Aging Eye*, *Living Well with Osteoarthritis*, and *Better Bladder and Bowel Control*—that provide more detailed information on treatments for the problems in this section. (For ordering information, see "Resources," page 51.)

Vestibular disorders

Ear infections, allergies, head injuries, or problems with blood circulation may temporarily or permanently affect the vestibular system in the inner ear. That sparks trouble with balance, dizziness, and vertigo (the sickening sensation that you or your surroundings are spinning). Treatment varies depending on the disorder. If dizziness and nausea are persistent, vestibular rehabilitation (balance retraining therapy) may be recommended. A trained vestibular rehabilita-

Good posture counts

Posture may not be the first thing that comes to mind when you're trying to improve your balance. But think back to when you were a child, playing with building blocks. They formed a more stable column if they were in an even line than if they were piled up haphazardly, with some of them off-center. The better the alignment, the less likely they were to topple.

So, too, with posture. Although your spine is not ramrod straight—it has a gentle, S-shaped curve that minimizes wear and tear and allows for greater flexibility—proper alignment of the spine and upper body are important for balance. Watch people walk, and you'll see how common it is for people to hold their bodies unevenly. If they trip, this can make it harder for them to catch their balance and avoid a fall.

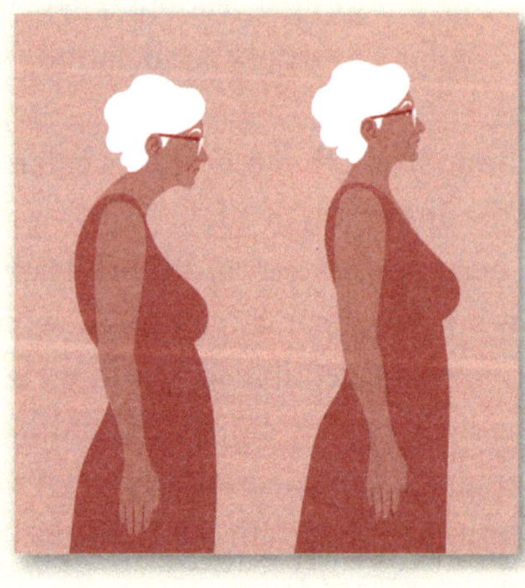

Poor posture can come from various causes, such as a lifetime of slouching, weakness in key muscle groups, or tightness in various muscles and tendons. As muscles tighten up, they shorten. This curtails range of motion—that is, how far a joint can move in a given direction—and it makes you less nimble. Unless you do stretches to counter this, your range of motion is likely to become increasingly limited.

Muscle strength matters for posture and balance, too. The so-called core muscles of the abdomen, back, side, pelvis, and buttocks are essential for holding yourself in proper alignment and making the microadjustments needed to stay steady. Strong back muscles are particularly important for counteracting slumping, which tips your body forward and thus off-center. Strong lower leg muscles are also important, to help keep you from swaying too much while standing.

The balance workouts in this report address these problems with exercises that build strength where it counts and with stretches that loosen tight muscles. Quick posture checks, ideally in front of a full-length mirror, will help. Here's what to aim for:

- chin parallel to the floor
- shoulders even (roll your shoulders up, back, and down to help find the correct position)
- ears in line with your shoulders
- neutral spine (no flexing or arching, only the spine's natural curves)
- arms at your sides with elbows even
- abdominal muscles pulled taut
- hips even
- shoulders in line with your hips
- knees even and pointing straight ahead
- feet pointing straight ahead
- body weight distributed evenly on both feet.

tion therapist can recommend a treatment plan combining certain head, body, and eye exercises, which may help ease these symptoms. Talk to your doctor about this.

Three common vestibular disorders pose particular problems with balance.

Benign paroxysmal positional vertigo (BPPV). Sometimes the tiny stones called canaliths tumble out of the utricle and into a semicircular canal (see "Vestibular system," page 3). The stones prevent the cupula and the sensory hair cells inside it from tilting properly, so that conflicting messages about the position of your head are sent to the brain. Turning your head to catch a glimpse behind you or rolling over in bed can cause the room-spinning sensation of vertigo. Possible causes of BPPV include head injury and aging. The Epley maneuver—a series of specific head movements done while you are sitting upright, then lying down—may help shift errant canaliths out of the semicircular canal. This canalith repositioning procedure must be guided by a trained clinician.

Labyrinthitis. When the labyrinth—the inner-ear structure containing the three semicircular canals, along with the utricle and saccule (see "Vestibular system," page 3)—is infected or swollen, temporary dizziness and loss of balance may occur. An upper respiratory tract ailment like tonsillitis, sinusitis, a cold, or an ear infection is often the culprit. Allergies, smoking, alcohol use, stress, and fatigue can increase the risk of developing labyrinthitis. Washing your hands often and getting an annual flu shot can help stave off certain infections that contribute to it.

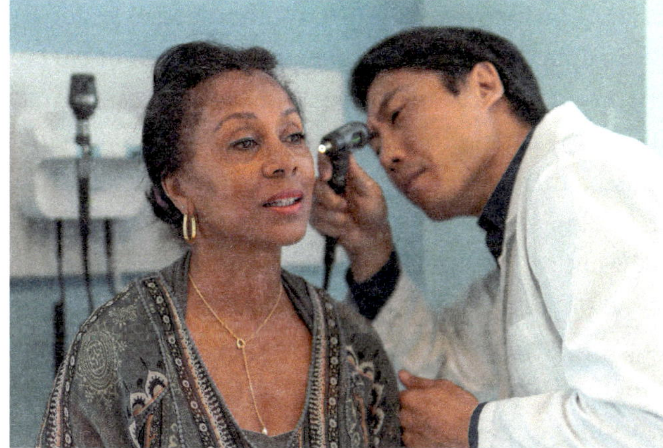

Ear infections or other ear problems may temporarily or permanently affect the vestibular system in the inner ear. Otolaryngologists (ear, nose, and throat doctors) specialize in treating these problems.

Ménière's disease. This condition, which typically strikes men and women between 20 and 50 years of age, affects both hearing and balance. Endolymph—the thick fluid inside the inner ear—builds up to the point where it ruptures the membranes that hold it, damaging the surrounding sensory cells. Spells of Ménière's disease come and go, lasting minutes or hours, and triggering hearing loss, vertigo, and tinnitus (persistent ringing or other noise in the ears). Sometimes this disorder stops on its own; in other cases, sufferers need medication or surgery for relief. Cutting down on salt (sodium) in your diet and limiting alcohol or caffeine can lessen the dizziness. Sometimes diuretic drugs help.

Eye disorders

Eye disorders can blur sight or punch holes in your field of vision, leading to balance problems and a higher fall risk. Four disorders are common culprits.

- Cataracts, which make your vision cloudy or blurry, are the most common of these problems. Older adults with cataracts are two to three times more likely to take a tumble than those without cataracts, but this eye disorder can now be easily corrected with minor surgery.
- Glaucoma initially diminishes peripheral vision, but if it's left untreated, it can lead to blindness. Because you might not notice changes in your vision at first, it's important to have regular eye exams as you age. You can prevent or reduce further damage with eye drops or surgery.
- Macular degeneration affects central vision before spreading outward. In addition, it causes distortion in vision, making straight lines appear wavy. Eventually, it can lead to blindness. Although the disease is not curable, early detection and treatment can minimize potential damage.
- Diabetic retinopathy can lead to blurred central vision and spots and floaters that create holes in the field of vision. Though there is no cure, various treatments—including laser therapies, medications that discourage the formation of new blood vessels, and steroids—can help prevent or slow vision loss.

Arthritis

Stiff, sore joints hamper movement. If your ankles or knees are arthritic, for example, it's hard to bend them, which affects your ability to balance and react when you trip. If your neck is stiff, your range of motion—how far you can move in any direction—is limited, so you tend to move your upper body to look behind you. This can upset your balance, too. Data show that people with painful knee or hip osteoarthritis fall 53% more often than those without arthritis, and up to 50% of people with arthritis fall in a year. The greater the number of joints affected, the bigger the risk.

Arthritis in the joints of the spine can also be a problem. If the arthritis becomes advanced, the space within the spinal column may narrow, as can the spaces between the bones, a condition that can cause pain, tingling, and numbness in the arms, legs, and back. You might keep your body stiff or adopt an awkward posture to avoid the pain and compensate for the numbness, but this can affect your balance, and a lack of exercise due to pain may lead to deconditioning, weak muscles, and ultimately falls.

Peripheral neuropathy

"Neuropathy" simply means nerve disease or damage, and "peripheral" means that the affected nerves are outside the central nervous system (the brain and spinal cord). Peripheral neuropathy may impede balance by impairing proprioception and muscle strength, as well as through the distracting quality of pain. Damaged motor or sensory nerves, for example, cause a variety of unpleasant symptoms, such as muscle weakness; shooting pains; burning; or numbness, tingling, and prickling sensations called paresthesias.

Often, nerve fibers farthest from the central nervous system—in the feet and legs, or hands and arms—malfunction first. Over 100 kinds of neuropathy have been identified. These ailments may be short-lived, lasting only until damaged nerves heal, or they may progress slowly and permanently.

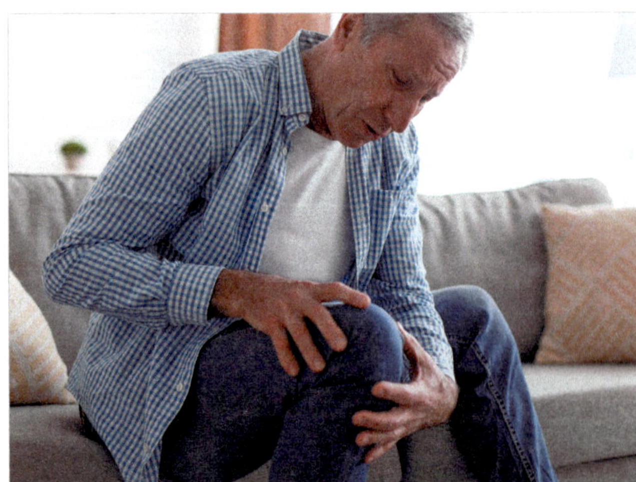

Stiff, sore joints hinder movement. If your ankles or knees are arthritic, for example, it's hard to bend them, which in turn affects your ability to balance and to react quickly when you trip.

Urinary incontinence

Having to get up in the middle of the night to urinate because of an overactive bladder may lead to falls or tripping over objects in the dark. Avoiding liquids in the evening and relieving yourself before bedtime may reduce the need to urinate overnight. Although many people are hesitant to speak about incontinence, you should talk with your doctor. In most cases, incontinence can be significantly improved with appropriate help, ranging from pelvic floor physical therapy to medications or surgery.

Heart arrhythmia

A change in the speed or rhythm of the heartbeat may interfere with blood supply to the brain, spurring sudden weakness or dizziness, or more serious problems like fainting or a heart attack.

Stroke

Strokes occur when a blocked blood vessel suddenly interrupts the flow of oxygen and nutrients to part of the brain, or, less often, when a blood vessel bursts inside the brain. The compromised brain cells die off, causing many serious problems that can affect balance, including weakness, numbness, trouble seeing, trouble walking, dizziness, and loss of coordination. Often, these physical deficits are confined to one side of the body. A stroke can wreak havoc on important mental functions that play into balance, including attention, working memory, and decision making. Stroke rehabilitation can be very effective at helping individuals regain their balance. It may not repair brain damage, but rehab exercises that target motor skills and mobility can help to reorganize and strengthen the elements of the balance control system that are still intact.

Microvascular disease in the brain

Just as some strokes can cause damaging bleeding into the brain, disease in the brain's small blood vessels can cause fluid leakage that harms white matter (the fatty tissue that insulates nerve fibers and facilitates communication between brain cells). This leads to brain changes that have been linked to gait and balance issues. The more severe the disease, the worse the problems with balance and gait.

Parkinson's disease

Cells in certain areas of the brain produce dopamine, a naturally occurring neurotransmitter that regulates movement, among other tasks. The loss of these brain cells causes Parkinson's disease, which affects the system of motor nerves throughout the body. This condition impairs balance in a variety of ways: through tremors in the legs and other parts of the body, rigidity of the limbs and trunk, slowness of movement called bradykinesia, and direct hindrance of systems affecting balance and coordination. Difficulty walking occurs as the disease progresses. General aerobic and strength training exercises are helpful. In addition, a form of non-contact boxing called Rock Steady Boxing has been found to improve balance, agility, speed, and strength in people with Parkinson's.

Multiple sclerosis

This unpredictable central nervous system condition disrupts communication between the brain and the body. It often causes muscle weakness and interferes with balance and coordination, sometimes making walking—or even standing—difficult or impossible. As multiple sclerosis advances, it can cause partial or complete paralysis. A variety of other possible symptoms may interfere with balance, too: dizziness, tremors, trouble with concentration and attention, and sensations of pain, numbness, prickling, or "pins and needles." As with Parkinson's, people with multiple sclerosis can often benefit from general aerobic and strength training exercises, performed at whatever level they are capable of doing safely.

Cognitive impairment and dementia

The ability to stand and walk is not just a simple, automatic motor function driven by your limbs and muscles, but rather a complex task that requires cognitive input. As such, declining mental and cognitive function can increase the risk for balance issues and falls because of impairments in attention, reaction time, decision making, detection of postural issues, and short-term memory. Yoga and tai chi can be helpful in preserving balance in people with dementia and cognitive impairment.

Medications that affect balance

By keeping blood sugar at safe levels, hearts thumping rhythmically, and moods afloat, medications can be lifesaving. Yet side effects and interactions between drugs (both prescription and nonprescription drugs) may increase your fall risk in numerous ways. For example, they can cause blurred vision, dizziness or lightheadedness stemming from low blood pressure, drowsiness, delirium, impaired alertness or judgment, and weakened muscles. Some medications may damage the inner ear, spurring temporary or permanent balance disorders.

Sometimes, problems stem from the sheer number of medicines you take, rather than a single drug. According to a national health survey, a third of 45- to 64-year-olds and two-thirds of people 65 and older take three or more prescription drugs over the course of a month. And 18% of 45- to 64-year-olds, as well as 42% of people 65 and over, take five or more drugs. Some gerontologists say they rarely see patients who take fewer than six or seven. Taking many medications at the same time can boost the severity and frequency of side effects among people of any age. Older adults are especially vulnerable, because people's bodies absorb and respond to drugs differently with age.

While it's true that some medicines are more likely to play a role in falls than others, many of these drugs are surprisingly difficult to avoid. A review published in *JAMA Internal Medicine* looked at medication use in a four-month period before and after a hip, shoulder, or wrist fracture among 168,133 Medicare beneficiaries. Before the fracture occurred, three-quarters of study participants had been taking at least one drug known to increase fall risk or decrease bone density, such as those described below. Yet only 7% of these patients stopped taking the problematic drugs after the fracture, while an equal proportion of patients started taking such drugs.

The list of drugs that increase fall risk includes but is not limited to the following:

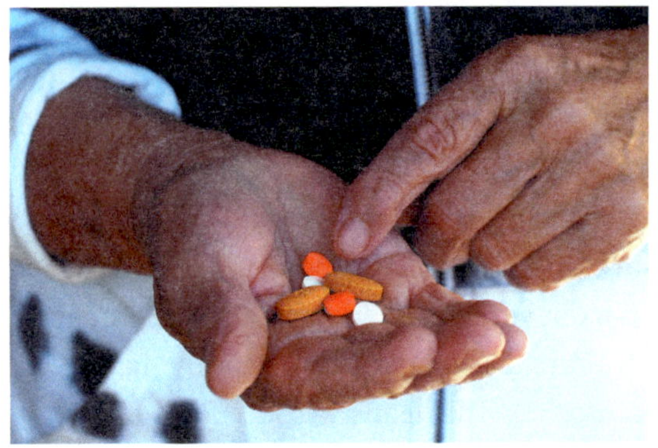

Review your medications with your doctor to see if any of them are contributing to balance problems. If so, ask if there are any pills you can eliminate or possibly swap for a less problematic alternative.

- antidepressant drugs, such as selective serotonin reuptake inhibitors (SSRIs) and serotonin-norepinephrine reuptake inhibitors (SNRIs)
- anti-anxiety drugs, such as benzodiazepines
- anticholinergic/antispasmodic drugs (used to treat stomach cramps)
- antihistamines
- blood pressure drugs, such as alpha blockers, centrally acting antihypertensives, ACE inhibitors, angiotensin-receptor blockers (ARBs), and beta blockers (including eye drops, which can lower blood pressure as a side effect)
- diabetes drugs, such as insulin, glipizide (Glucotrol), and glyburide (DiaBeta, others)
- heart drugs, such as anti-arrhythmics, nitrates and other vasodilators, and digoxin
- pain drugs, such as opioids, nonsteroidal anti-inflammatory drugs (NSAIDs), and gabapentin (Neurontin)
- sleep drugs, such as sedatives and hypnotics.

Generally, it's wise to keep the number of medications you take to a minimum. Routinely discuss your medications with your doctor to ensure this.

How your doctor can help

If you are experiencing side effects that could make falls more likely, ask your primary care doctor or gerontologist to do a medication review. Put all your prescription and nonprescription medications and supplements into a bag and bring them with you to this visit—or at least bring a complete and up-to-date list, including how much you take of each and when you take it. It's best to carry such a list with you at all times, anyway, in case of an emergency. For the purposes of the review, however, it's likely to be more accurate if you bring everything with you, as people tend to leave things off the list, especially supplements and the doses they take.

Your doctor may consider various strategies, such as the following, to reduce drug-related fall risks.

Prune the list. Medications tend to multiply, especially if you see several doctors. One specialist may put you on a drug, unaware that another physician has prescribed a similar drug—or perhaps one that causes an adverse interaction. Your doctor can review the list to make sure you still need these drugs and get rid of any you don't need.

Consider a lower dose. This can be especially helpful for reducing side effects from diuretics and heart drugs. Your doctor can determine whether it is safe to change a dose. Don't try this on your own.

Substitute a drug. Sometimes it's possible to switch to a drug with different side effects.

Change the time of day a drug is taken. For example, taking all your blood pressure medications first thing in the morning may cause your blood pressure to drop too low, increasing your risk of falls. Your doctor might suggest that you separate your blood pressure pills, taking some in the morning and some in the evening.

Make lifestyle changes. Sometimes, changes in your daily routine work well enough to enable you to lower the dose of a medication or eliminate it entirely. You might be able to apply relaxation techniques and sleep hygiene tips that allow you to safely taper off sleep medication, for instance. Or you might improve your diet and exercise routine enough that the doctor can lower your doses of diabetes and blood pressure drugs. Weight loss alone can often reduce or eliminate the need for blood pressure and diabetes pills.

Safety measures to prevent falls

Occasional scrapes, bangs, and bruises from falls are a fact of life from childhood onward. Consequences grow worse as you age, however. Among people 65 and older, falling ranks as the top cause of injuries. Every year, millions of nonfatal injuries are serious enough to merit a trip to the hospital emergency department. The safety measures in this chapter will help you skirt problems by addressing any health risks you may have and by "fall-proofing" your home.

Why do people fall?

Often, falls occur when multiple risk factors collide. Some risks are extrinsic, meaning that they have to do with the environment around you—for example, broken pavement, a slick area of ice or wet floor, clutter, dim lighting that hides obstacles, the rolled edge of a rug, or a curb you didn't notice. Others are intrinsic—that is, specific to you. These might include vision trouble; declining muscle strength, power, and flexibility; any health problem or medication that affects balance; a low level of confidence in your balance; or a fear of falling (see page 14). To prevent falls, then, it makes sense to address both types of problems.

The U.S. Preventive Services Task Force (USPSTF) has found that the most promising strategy for addressing intrinsic issues is exercise. In a review of 62 studies, the USPSTF correlated exercise with an 11% reduction in the number of people falling and a 19% reduction in "injurious" falls. According to a 2020 review of 116 studies by the Cochrane Collaboration (an international organization that conducts reviews of medical literature), the most effective exercise programs for fall prevention are ones that incorporate both balance work and functional exercises (exercises that mimic everyday activities)—exactly what you'll find in this report.

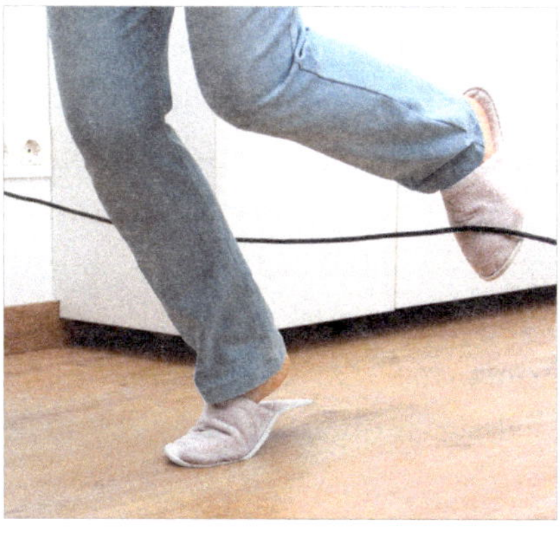

If your house is typical, it might as well be booby-trapped. Most contain numerous tripping hazards like throw rugs, power cords, and clutter (including shoes) on the floor.

There are no clinical trials testing extrinsic strategies, but certainly, clearing clutter from the floor, installing grab rails in the shower, tying shoelaces properly, and similar safety measures remain wise (see "Home safety checklist," page 17). However, you cannot always control extrinsic factors, such as the weather. If it's icy and snowy outside, try to avoid going out. If you must go out, try putting inexpensive ice cleats (like Stabilicers or Yaktrax) on your shoes—or walk like a penguin (see "Icy out? Try walking like a penguin," page 15.)

Personal safety checklist

As an old adage tells us, an ounce of prevention is worth a pound of cure. Scan this list for any problems that raise your risk for falls. Then take action to solve problems one by one. Balance training, which is covered in the workouts in this report, is a big part of the solution, too.

Eye problems

Eyesight less than 20/60, decreasing depth perception, and reduced sensitivity to contrast—all of which can be detected in a standard eye exam—contribute to falls. So do eye disorders like cataracts, glaucoma, macular degeneration, and diabetic retinopathy, which impair your vision (see "Eye disorders," page 9).

Fixes: Have your eyes tested annually to detect any new problems (or more often, if you have a progressive eye disorder). Discuss options for correcting your vision. Install appropriately bright lighting at home.

The wrong eyewear

Reading glasses, bifocals, trifocals, and progressive lenses are enormously helpful in correcting vision, but they can be hazardous when you're walking. If you look straight ahead as you walk, these lenses blur objects scattered on the floor or ground, making it hard to see possible hazards.

Fixes: Save reading glasses for close work only—not walking. Consider buying a pair of glasses with single-vision distance lenses for activities like walking outdoors. If you do choose to wear bifocals, trifocals, or progressive lenses, be careful to look through the appropriate section of the lenses while walking. Talk to an eye specialist about your options.

Poor posture

Poor posture can throw your body off balance.

Fixes: Try to stand up straight. Check your posture whenever you're in front of a mirror (see "Good posture counts," page 8). The stretches and core strength exercises in this report can help, too.

Weak muscles

Loss of strength and power—particularly in the lower body—erodes balance, setting the stage for falls and making it hard to catch yourself if you trip. Tight muscles limit range of motion.

Fixes: Exercise can improve strength, power, reflexes, and balance, while stretches enhance flexibility. Get the exercise you need to stay strong and healthy through balance workouts, walk-

Fear of falling

Fear of falling is widespread among older people. While normal caution is beneficial, the fear of falling can actually lead to harm. For example, some people pull back entirely from a range of activities that are still well within their abilities, precipitating a downward spiral in which reduced activity leads to physical deconditioning and worse balance, along with a poorer quality of life in general. Other people continue their activities but stiffen their bodies when doing something they perceive as risky, such as walking on an uneven path. By stiffening up, they may diminish their ability to respond quickly to a stumble. Moreover, the cognitive demands of dealing with this fear can take away from brain resources that are needed to preserve balance.

What can help ease the fear of falling?

There are a couple of practices that appear to help. At the top of the list is tai chi, a form of exercise that involves moving gently through a series of poses in a controlled fashion. Multiple clinical trials have shown that it can significantly lower the risk of falling when practiced regularly. And in a randomized clinical trial of 60 adults ages 60 and older, participants who did tai chi three times a week for eight weeks decreased their fear of falling. With such encouraging findings, researchers at the Oregon Research Institute, under a grant from the federal government, developed a program called Tai Chi: Moving for Better Balance. The program has demonstrated effectiveness in reducing fall risk and improving balance and physical performance among people ages 70 and older. Importantly, it has also been shown to help reduce the fear of falling. The program is available in communities across the country. Check with your local Y.

Similarly, yoga in a group setting has been shown in small studies to help reduce the fear of falling, but it's important to go to classes that are appropriate to your age and ability level so you don't feel overwhelmed or get injured.

ing, and other activities described in this report.

Stiff, sore joints

Stiff joints limit movement and make it harder to catch yourself if you do trip. If you have trouble turning your neck, for example, you tend to turn your upper body to look behind you, which can throw you off balance. Pain itself takes attention away from walking or moving safely (see "Pain and falls," page 16). Because it may be painful to walk, you may move less, which over time will contribute to further pain, muscle loss, and stiffness. Excess weight increases the risk of painful knee arthritis.

Fixes: Discuss ways to ease painful, swollen joints with your doctor. Strengthening exercises and stretches will help, too, according to the Arthritis Foundation. If you are overweight, try to lose weight.

Weak ankles

Weak ankles or stiff, inflexible ankle joints make walking harder. Stumbles may occur more when the rear foot doesn't clear the ground properly, making the toes more likely to catch against the ground as you move forward.

Fixes: Stretches and strengthening exercises shown in the balance workouts in this report will help.

Foot pain

Foot pain or numbness may make falls more likely.

Fixes: Discuss options for easing pain with your doctor. Call your doctor if you notice pain, burning, or numbness in your feet. Your doctor can help treat a variety of painful conditions.

Unstable shoes

High heels, slip-on shoes, loose slippers, and smooth, slippery soles may promote falls.

Fixes: Wear sturdy shoes, preferably with low or flat heels and nonskid, rubber soles. Avoid wearing just socks. Shoes or sneakers with Velcro closures are good bets to prevent you from tripping on laces.

Chronic diseases

Blood pressure fluctuations, heart problems, inner ear disorders, and nerve damage are among the ailments that contribute to falls (see "Health conditions that affect balance," page 8).

Fixes: Consult your doctor if you suffer from dizziness or other balance problems.

Medications

Many medications cause dizziness or drowsiness that can precede a fall (see "Medications that affect balance," page 11).

Fixes: Report dizziness or drowsiness to your doctor. Discuss whether changing medications or lowering dosages might help. Bring medications and supplements (or a list detailing them) to doctor's visits. It is helpful to keep notes on when dizziness occurs to see if it is related to when you take your medicines.

Alcohol use

Alcohol impairs judgment, slows reaction time, and cranks up clumsiness—a veritable recipe for falls. Worse, as people age, it takes less alcohol to prompt such problems. Mixing medications and alcohol can

Icy out? Try walking like a penguin

Penguins walk on ice all the time. They're experts at it, so follow their lead and walk like a penguin. Here's why. When you walk normally, your weight shifts from the ball of your back foot to the heel of your front foot. During this transition, neither foot is flat on the ground, so you are inherently less stable and therefore more likely to fall—especially if your front heel slides out from under you, which can easily happen if the forward foot fails to gain traction on an icy patch.

Instead, the next time you're on an icy sidewalk, turn out your feet slightly and take short, flat-footed steps, keeping your feet underneath you rather than extending your front leg forward. This way your feet stay in greater contact with the ground, and your center of gravity is more stable, reducing your risk of falling. Be sure to keep your hands out of your pockets to help you catch your balance if needed.

Pain and falls

Pain is a constant companion for people who live with arthritis, low back problems, or other chronic ailments. It can also upset your balance.

Using data gathered for the MOBILIZE Boston study, which followed 749 adults ages 65 or older for close to three years, researchers considered the role that pain plays in falls. For a year and a half, participants completed monthly calendar cards, marking down whether they had fallen and the average amount of pain they had felt during that month. During the study period, 55% of participants fell at least once. Writing in *JAMA*, the researchers reported that falls were more common among those who complained of two or more painful sites on the body or more severe pain at the start of the trial. Use of pain relievers did not change the risk of falling in this study. More recent research shows that the risk of falling may double if you suffer from pain in multiple sites.

Pain may contribute to falls in multiple ways—by weakening muscles, fostering muscle imbalances, slowing nerve and muscle responses, creating a distraction, or derailing mental resources like attention that would normally help a person avoid a fall or recover from a stumble. Here are steps to ease pain and reduce your risk of falling:

Work with your doctor to control pain better. Choosing the right type and level of pain medication may require some trial and error. Be aware of any dizziness or drowsiness from drugs, and report these symptoms to your doctor.

Seek ways to reduce pain other than medication. Acupuncture shows promise in easing chronic low back pain and osteoarthritis pain in the knees. Gentle self-massage and applications of cold or heat may help, although this depends on the underlying problem causing your pain. Explore these and other options with your doctor to find an approach that fits your situation.

Exercise. Physical activity can help reduce some forms of chronic pain. However, you may need to avoid repetitive or jarring movements, such as running or even too much walking. Water aerobics, tai chi, gentle forms of yoga (see the Yoga Balance Workout, page 32), and low-impact exercises (see the Beginner Balance Workout, page 26) may be better choices. If your pain results from arthritis, try the two-hour pain rule recommended by the Arthritis Foundation. Realize that some short-lived discomfort is likely when you exercise, especially if you haven't been active. However, if you feel more pain two hours after you finish exercising than before you started, you probably overdid it. Pare back till this is no longer true (for example, by walking less or doing fewer reps or sets of exercises). Then, step up your level of exercise very gradually, keeping the rule in mind.

Be sure your footwear is as comfortable and supportive as possible. Adding cushions for tender spots and orthotics to properly position your feet may help. See a podiatrist, if necessary.

If you do suffer from chronic pain, be aware that it is a powerful distraction. It could make you more likely to slip or trip in unknown, uneven, or dimly lit surroundings. So, good lighting, clearing away obstacles, and trying to focus attention when walking are especially important for you.

exacerbate side effects like dizziness or drowsiness. Additionally, alcohol raises the risk for developing the inner ear disorders labyrinthitis and Ménière's disease (see "Vestibular disorders," page 8). Alcoholism is also one cause of peripheral neuropathy, which also affects balance.

Fixes: Avoid or limit alcohol. This is especially important if you take medication or have labyrinthitis or Ménière's disease. If you do drink, be aware of how alcohol affects you.

Excess weight

Excess weight can cause gait problems that may affect your center of balance. Being overweight or obese also puts painful strain on your knees and hips. (Just walking across level ground requires the knees to support up to one-and-a-half times your body weight; when going up or down stairs, each knee bears two to three times your body weight.) In addition, it increases your risk for developing osteoarthritis of the knee, which in turn can cause changes in gait as well as sudden pain that can make you lurch or lose your balance. Being overweight also increases the risk of diabetes, which can lead to neuropathy in your feet that can affect balance.

Fixes: You can reduce pressure on the knee by strengthening the quadriceps muscles on the front of your thighs through regular balance workouts and daily walks, if possible. Better yet, try to reach a healthier weight by combining these workouts with a healthy diet.

Home safety checklist

Improving your balance is a great way to prevent falls, but you should also do an annual room-by-room safety inventory of your home to spot tripping hazards. There are simple fixes for most of these problems. By reviewing this list periodically, you can make updates as your needs change.

Bedrooms

- ☐ Keep a phone and lamp close to your bed. Lamps that turn on at a touch or by sound are easy to manage, so you don't fumble in the dark.
- ☐ A firm mattress helps with balance as you rise from the bed. Make sure the bed is low enough that you can put your feet flat on the floor when you're sitting on the edge.
- ☐ Arrange furniture so that the path to the door is clear.
- ☐ If you use a cane or walker, keep it within easy reach when you go to bed.

Bathrooms

- ☐ Install night lights.
- ☐ Install grab bars and nonslip mats or adhesive safety strips in the bathtub or shower.
- ☐ If you have trouble sitting down on the toilet or getting up from it, install an elevated seat with armrests or an elevated "comfort height" toilet.
- ☐ If the floor is slippery when wet, consider installing textured tiles to help prevent falls.
- ☐ If tub height is a problem, consider installing a low-threshold shower or a walk-in tub.

Kitchen

- ☐ Store often-used items where you can easily reach them.
- ☐ Keep a sturdy step stool handy to reach items in high cabinets.

Entrances and hallways

- ☐ All outside doors should have lights.
- ☐ Keep outside walkways free of cracks, holes, and clutter.
- ☐ Repair any rotted or crumbling steps.
- ☐ Mats inside the door should lie flat and have a nonskid backing.
- ☐ Hallways should be well lit.

Stairways

- ☐ Make sure there is a light switch at the top and bottom of the stairway.

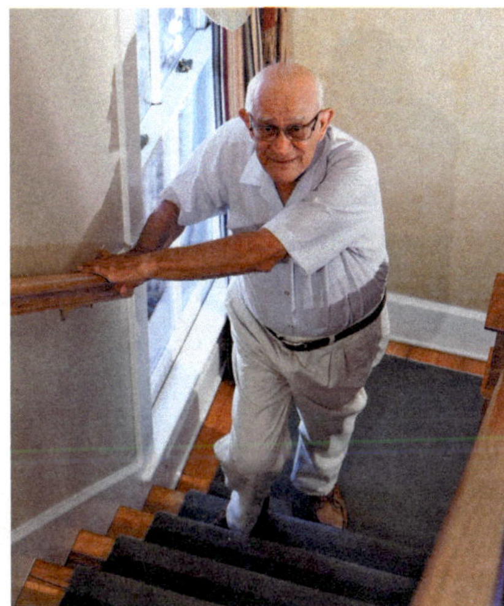

Keep stairs in good repair and free of clutter. Stair carpeting, if any, should be tacked down tightly.

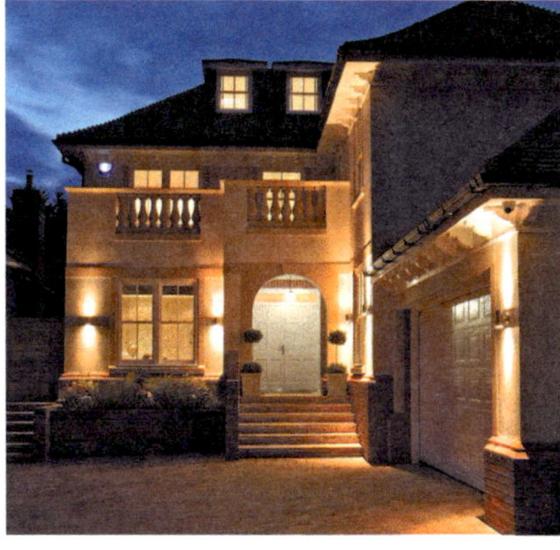

Good lighting throughout the home is important. Exterior doors should also be well lit, particularly if you have steps there.

- ☐ Install a handrail that runs the full length of the stairs, preferably on both sides of the stairs.
- ☐ Keep stairs in good repair and clear of clutter.
- ☐ Stair carpeting, if any, should be tacked down tightly.

Housewide

- ☐ Keep floors clutter-free.
- ☐ Keep electric cords tucked out of the way.
- ☐ Make sure you can turn on lights without walking into rooms.
- ☐ Lighting should be even, with no splashes of shadow or glare. Add task lights where needed.
- ☐ Skip scatter rugs, if possible. All carpeting should lie flat and have nonskid backing.
- ☐ Program emergency numbers into phones.
- ☐ If door thresholds create tripping hazards, replace them with lower thresholds (a quarter-inch if edges are square, or a half-inch if edges are slanted).

Activities that enhance balance

The workouts in this report are designed to improve your balance skills, both while you hold steady (static balance) and while you're in motion (dynamic balance). Standing with one foot in front of another, lifting a foot off the floor, and shifting your weight in various directions are examples of simple balance exercises you can sprinkle throughout your day. In addition, experts at the American College of Sports Medicine suggest ways you can pose balance challenges for yourself.

- **Reduce your base of support.** Instead of standing on two legs hip-width apart, stand with your feet together, and then stand on one leg. This makes you work harder to stabilize yourself, relying more on your core muscles and less on a broad base of support to maintain your balance.
- **Shift your center of gravity.** Even something as simple as walking requires continual readjustments to stay steady. If you walk forward putting one foot directly in front of the other, as you would on a balance beam, this combines two challenges—a narrow base of support and movement.
- **Switch from a flat, stable surface to a soft, rounded, or otherwise less stable, more irregular surface.** The lack of predictability forces you to pay greater attention to every movement and strengthens circuits in the brain that govern balance.
- **Close your eyes.** Visual input plays a role in proprioception. If you stand on one leg with your eyes closed, you'll find it's much harder than with your eyes open. (Keep a chair nearby to steady yourself.)

Certain types of exercise are particularly good at building balance skills or the strength and flexibility that underlie good balance. If you're active, you likely practice some of these already. The following list may suggest others you would like to try.

- **Walking, biking, and climbing stairs** strengthen muscles in your lower body, which are essential for balance because they provide your base of support. (Using a recumbent bike or stair stepper is an option if your balance is compromised.)
- **Hiking** takes the balance challenges of walking up a notch, adding issues like uneven ground, slopes, rocks, roots, and streams.
- **Resistance exercise** (weight training) builds muscles. Many of the strengthening exercises in our workouts focus on hip and leg muscles. Some back and abdominal muscles are targeted, too, to help improve posture and balance.
- **Core exercises** build stabilizing muscles that help keep you upright and prevent a trip from turning into a fall (see "Three exercises to improve core strength," page 19).
- **Stretches** ease tight muscles, improving posture and balance (see "Good posture counts," page 8).
- **Yoga** strengthens and stretches tight muscles, while challenging static and dynamic balance. There are many styles of yoga and many ways to modify the poses to suit your own ability. Regular practice yields the most benefit. Our Yoga Balance Workout (page 32) and Advanced Yoga Balance Workout (page 43) offer a variety of classic poses.
- **Tai chi** hones balance with a combination of slow, choreographed moves, gradual shifts of weight from one foot to another, rotation of the trunk, and extension of the limbs. It is a low-intensity form of exercise that has been shown in multiple studies to help improve balance, coordination, flexibility, muscle strength, and stamina. Correct posture and deep breathing are key elements of the practice.
- **Pilates** is an exercise program developed by Joseph Pilates in the 1920s that directly targets and strengthens your core muscles, while improving posture and flexibility. Certain exercises are designed to challenge static and dynamic balance.
- **Sports like pickleball, table tennis, and golf** help balance skills by making you constantly adjust your center of balance. In addition, they strengthen lower-

body muscles (assuming you're walking from hole to hole in golf, rather than hopping into a golf cart).

For all these forms of exercise, regular practice is key. What if you're not active at all? Take heart. Research shows that even people who have been sedentary can dramatically improve strength and balance through exercise, regardless of age. Our balance workouts will show you how to make gains safely.

Three exercises to improve core strength

Having strong abdominal, back, side, pelvic, and buttock muscles—what's known as your core—helps you maintain a healthy back and good posture and, as a result, improves your balance. Strong core muscles underlie almost everything you do, from walking to playing sports. That's because your core forms the sturdy central link between your upper and lower body. Forces that propel movement either originate in your core or else transfer through it on the way from one part of the body to another. Pilates and yoga routines can strengthen your core, as can the three moves shown here, which you can add to any of the balance routines you select.

1 | Opposite arm and leg raise

Starting position: Kneel on all fours, knees hip-width apart. Align your shoulders over your wrists and your hips over your knees. Keep your head and spine in alignment.

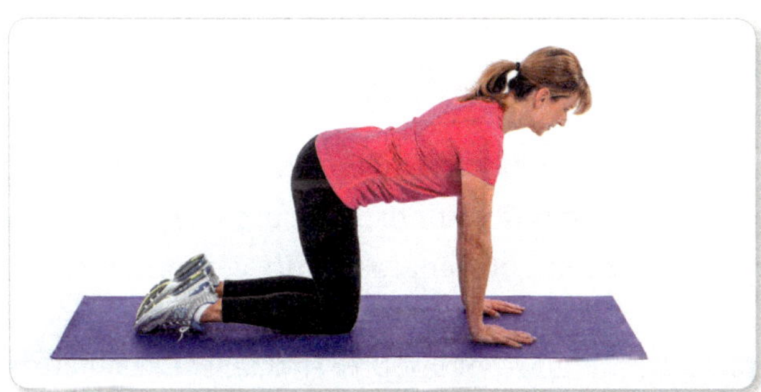

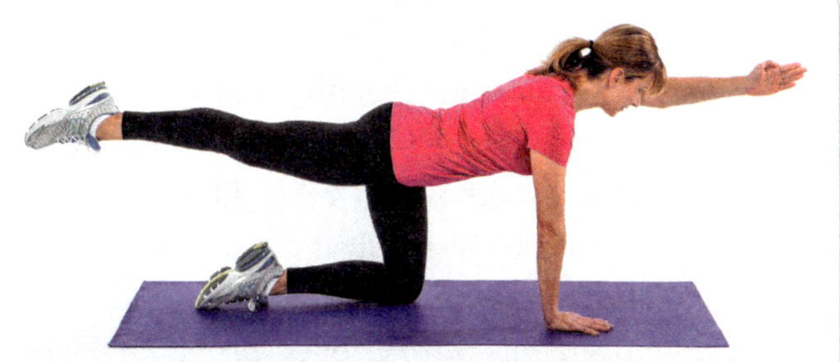

Movement: Extend your right leg off the floor behind you while reaching your left arm out in front of you. Try to raise your extended leg and arm parallel to the floor. Hold for 10 to 30 seconds. Return to the starting position, then repeat with your left leg and right arm. Do this two to four times on each side. Rest 30 to 90 seconds and repeat the entire set.

2 | Bridge

Starting position: Lie on your back with your knees bent and feet flat on the floor, hip-width apart. Place your arms at your sides. Relax your shoulders against the floor.

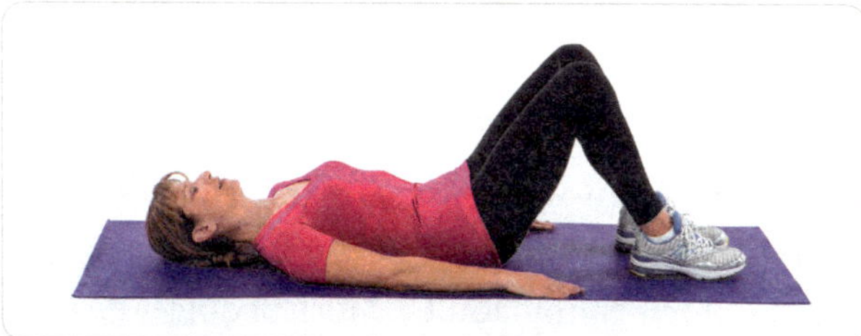

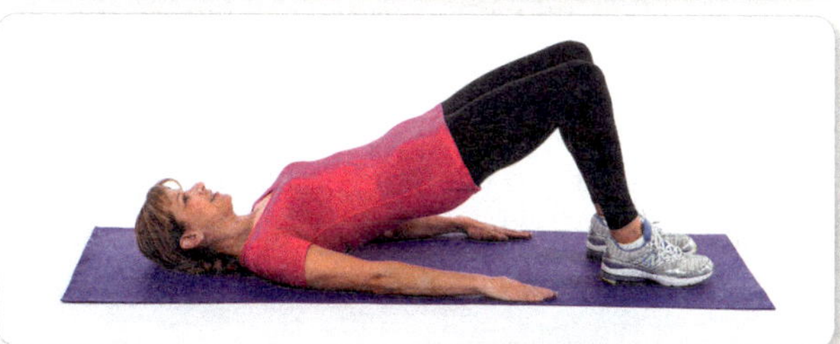

Movement: Tighten your abdominal muscles and your buttocks, press your heels into the floor, and lift your hips off the floor as high as is comfortable, or until they are in line with your shoulders and knees. Keep your hips even and spine neutral. Hold for a second. Return to the starting position. Do this eight to 12 times. Rest 30 to 90 seconds and repeat the entire set.

3 | Plank

Starting position: Begin on your hands and knees.

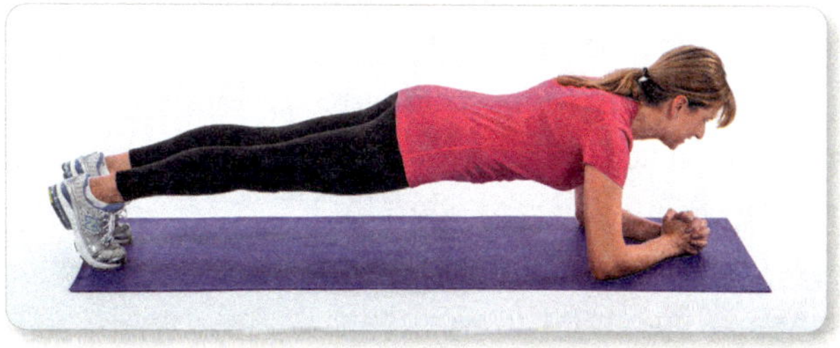

Movement: Tighten your abdominal muscles and lower your upper body onto your forearms, with your hands clasped and your elbows directly under your shoulders. Extend both legs with your feet flexed and toes touching the floor, so that you balance your body in a line like a plank. Hold for 15 to 60 seconds. Rest 30 to 90 seconds and repeat one to three times.

Starting balance workouts safely

Our program aims to help you become steadier on your feet. But before starting the workouts, consider whether you need to call your doctor for a go-ahead or see another expert who can help you work on your balance safely.

Do you need to see a doctor?

As every physician will tell you, exercise is essential for a healthy life. Generally, light to moderate exercise is safe for healthy adults. Most people—healthy or not—can safely take up walking. But before starting our walking program or the balance workouts, it's best to check in with your doctor if

- you feel unsteady on your feet or are afraid of falling
- you have dizzy spells or take medicine that makes you feel dizzy or drowsy
- you have a chronic or unstable health condition, such as heart disease (or several risk factors for heart disease), asthma or another respiratory ailment, high blood pressure, osteoporosis, or diabetes
- you have joint pain or musculoskeletal problems such as back, knee, or shoulder issues, including a herniated disc.

If you are uncertain, you may want to assess your risk for falling. The CDC offers a simple checklist that can help you do that. You can download it at www.health.harvard.edu/prevent-falls. Another useful tool is the Get Active Questionnaire developed by the Canadian Society for Exercise Physiology. You can find it at www.health.harvard.edu/GAQ.

If your risk is high, you should talk to your doctor before starting the workouts in this report. Ask if you can follow the specific balance workouts you'd like to try from this report. The Beginner Balance Workout (page 26) is an easy entry point for practically anyone, no matter what age. Odds are good that your doctor will feel the easier workouts and walking plan are fine as long as you start gradually, build up slowly, and attend to safety tips—including using a cane or walker, if you normally use one. Or, possibly, your doctor might want to modify certain exercises. If necessary, your doctor can refer you to a physiatrist, physical therapist, or another specialist like a neurologist or cardiologist for further evaluation. Sometimes, it's safest to work out with the supervision of an experienced personal trainer or a health professional, or to attend a supervised class at a hospital or other facility.

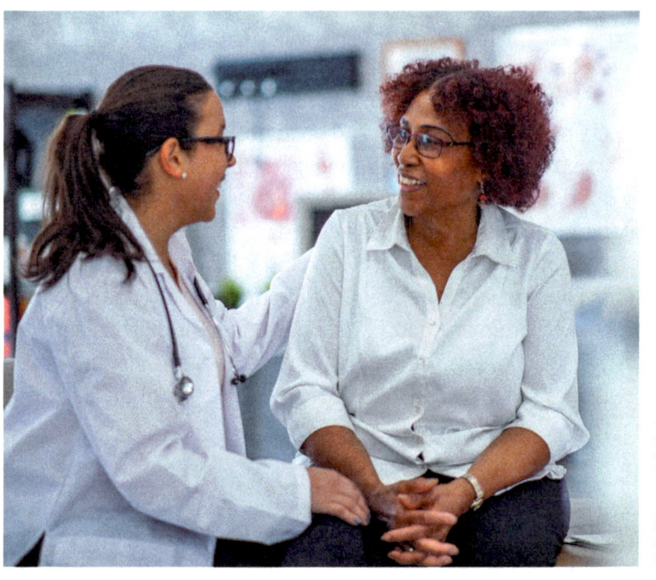

Light to moderate exercise is generally safe for healthy adults. But if you feel unsteady on your feet or are afraid of falling, talk with your physician before starting an exercise program.

Physiatrists, also known as rehabilitation physicians, are board-certified medical doctors who specialize in treating nerve, muscle, and bone conditions that affect movement. Stroke, back problems, Parkinson's disease, neuropathy, and debilitating arthritis or obesity are a few examples. A physiatrist can tailor exercises to enhance recovery after surgery or an injury, or work with limitations posed by pain or problems affecting movement. He or she can also tell you whether certain types of exercise will be helpful or harmful given your specific health history.

Physical therapists help restore abilities to people with health problems or injuries affecting muscles, bones, or nerves. Their expertise can be valuable if you have suffered a lingering sprain or are recovering from a stroke or heart attack. Some specialize in geriatrics, orthopedics, cardiopulmonary rehabilitation, or other areas. After having received a bachelor's degree, physical therapists must graduate from an accredited physical therapy program. Most of these programs offer doctoral degrees. Additionally, physical therapists must pass a national exam given by the Federation of State Boards of Physical Therapy and be licensed by their state. Those who specialize complete advanced training and additional national exams to become board certified.

Physical therapy assistants provide physical therapy services under the supervision of a physical therapist. They must complete a two-year associate's degree, pass a national exam, and, in most states, be licensed.

Personal trainers are fitness specialists who can help ensure that you're doing exercises properly. While encouraging and motivating you, they can teach you new skills, fine-tune your form, change up routines to beat boredom, and safely push you to the next level. But it's important to find a good one. No nationwide licensing requirements exist for personal trainers, although standards for the accrediting fitness organizations that train them have been set by the National Commission for Certifying Agencies. Two well-respected organizations that offer programs of study for personal trainers are the American College of Sports Medicine and the American Council on Exercise. Others include the National Council on Strength and Fitness, the National Strength and Conditioning Association, and the National Academy of Sports Medicine. All fitness organizations have different requirements for training and expertise. Some trainers specialize in working with particular populations—for example, older adults or athletes—and may have taken courses and possibly certifying exams in these areas.

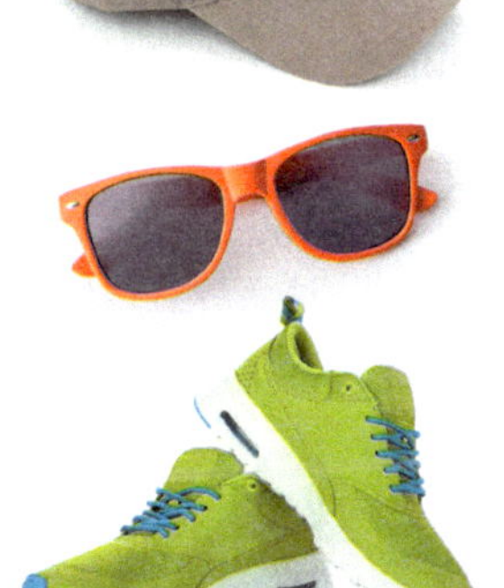

Proper gear is important—most notably, well-padded shoes. If you're exercising outdoors, dress for the weather. That means layers if you're going out in the cold, or a hat, sunscreen, sunglasses, and water bottle if it's warm out.

Top to bottom: © DonNichols, © Kubra Cavus, © talevr | Getty Images

Additional safety tips

The following tips can help you use the workouts in this report safely.

Pay attention. If your attention is focused, you'll be less likely to fall.

Stay steady. If you regularly use a cane or walker, use it during the exercises, too. If not, you can steady yourself with a sturdy chair or counter, or by standing in a corner of the room. If you feel dizzy while exercising, sit down until the feeling passes.

Do the warm-ups. Prepare your body for the workout by following the instructions in "Warm-ups" on page 25.

Go slow. Hurrying or pushing yourself too hard can cause accidents. Initially, less is better: consider doing fewer repetitions or an easier variation of an exercise the first time you try it.

Engage your core. Practice tightening your abdominal muscles as you stand or sit up straight. Imagine that you are preparing to counter a push from the front, side, or back. When you do balance exercises, you'll use this skill to help keep your balance.

Wear the right outfit. Choose comfortably padded sneakers or walking shoes with rubber soles. If you'll be walking outside (see "A walking plan," page 23), wear layers in cool weather, plus a hat, sunscreen, and sunglasses, as needed.

Drink water. Dehydration contributes to dizziness, weakness, heart rhythm disturbances, and low blood pressure. Throughout the day and before exercising, make sure you drink enough water to stay hydrated. Sip water during workouts and walks, too. If you find this means you need a bathroom break, take it before you have to hurry. A fall may be more likely when you're in a rush.

Don't forget to stretch. It's easy to ignore stretching at the end of a workout, but stretching helps prevent stiffness and keeps you limber (see "Finish with stretches," page 47).

Balance workouts and your overall fitness plan

Better balance is important. But to maintain your overall health, you need to do more than just balance exercises. You need to engage in physical activity on a regular basis. This chapter offers insight into current exercise guidelines and the benefits of exercise.

Current exercise recommendations

The Physical Activity Guidelines for Americans from the U.S. Department of Health and Human Services outline the types and amounts of exercise you should be doing to help maintain your health.

- All adults—including people with disabilities—should aim for a total of 150 minutes of moderate aerobic activity a week, or 75 minutes of vigorous activity, or an equivalent mix of the two. (Twenty minutes of moderate activity is roughly equal to 10 minutes of vigorous activity.) During moderate activity, you can talk, but not sing; during vigorous activity, you can manage only a few words aloud without pausing to breathe. You can gain additional health benefits by increasing your weekly total to 300 minutes of moderate activity, or 150 minutes of vigorous activity, or a mix.
- Strengthening exercises for all major muscle groups (legs, hips, back, abdomen, chest, shoulders, and arms) are recommended, too. Aim for two or more sessions per week, with 48 hours between sessions to let muscles recover.
- Balance exercises are recommended for older adults at risk of falling. But that doesn't mean they're not of great benefit for younger adults, too, to prevent accidents and improve athletic performance.
- Flexibility exercises may be helpful.

If this much activity isn't possible for you, experts suggest doing as much as you can. Some activity is always better than none. Even short bursts of activity, such as five or 10 minutes of walking several times a day, are helpful. As the guidelines say, the overall goal is to "move more and sit less." A tracking device such as a Fitbit or a simple pedometer can help you monitor how much exercise you're getting and can motivate you to meet exercise goals.

The health benefits of exercise

Meeting the exercise guidelines can help you feel, think, and look better. Evidence from thousands of studies shows that engaging in regular exercise

- tacks years onto your life
- helps prevent falls that can lead to debilitating fractures and loss of independence
- lowers your risks for early death, heart disease, stroke, diabetes, high blood pressure, and metabolic syndrome (a complex problem that blends three or more of the following factors: high blood pressure, high triglycerides, low "good" HDL cholesterol, a large waistline, and difficulty regulating blood sugar)
- promotes cardiovascular health in numerous ways—by improving your balance of blood lipids (increasing "good" HDL while lowering "bad" LDL cholesterol and triglycerides), which in turn helps prevent plaque buildup; helping arteries stay resilient despite aging; bumping up the number of blood vessels feeding the heart; reducing inflammation; and discouraging the formation of blood clots that can block coronary arteries
- lessens the likelihood of getting a variety of types of cancer, including colon, breast, lung, esophageal, endometrial, and stomach cancer
- helps keep you from gaining weight
- helps lessen abdominal obesity, which plays a role in many serious ailments, including heart disease, diabetes, and stroke
- eases depression
- boosts mental sharpness in older adults and may lower the risk of Alzheimer's disease
- improves the ability of older adults to carry out

everyday activities such as climbing stairs, hefting groceries, or getting up from a chair
- boosts bone density (provided the exercises are weight-bearing, meaning they work against gravity)
- lowers the risk for hip fractures
- promotes better sleep.

Fitting balance workouts into an overall exercise plan

Both the balance workouts and the walking plan outlined below are part of your balance training. The walking plan can also help you fulfill your aerobic activity requirements. It ramps up slowly and safely. By week 8, you'll meet the guidelines for aerobic exercise, assuming you can handle the increasing challenges.

Aim to do the balance workout you've chosen two to three times a week. Our workouts emphasize exercises that strengthen legs, hips, and certain core muscles. Stretches help with flexibility. And, of course, every workout focuses on enhancing balance.

So, by following our routine you'll be meeting most of the requirements in the U.S. exercise guidelines. Additional exercises to strengthen your chest, back, abdominal muscles, arms, and shoulders will help you meet the twice-weekly strength exercise recommendation. If you're not sure which strength exercises to add, see the "Resources" section (page 51) for other Harvard Medical School Special Health Reports that discuss strength training.

A walking plan: Simple steps to better balance

Building lower-body strength helps improve balance. Walks can help you do so safely, and they count toward your aerobic activity goals. If health problems make walks especially difficult for you, discuss your options with a physiatrist or physical therapist. Swimming or using specific exercise machines may be a better choice.

Our walking plan is designed to safely boost physical activity whether you're sedentary or fairly active. The minutes count, not the miles. Here's how to tailor the plan to your needs.

If you aren't in the habit of exercising: Start at the beginning, with Week 1. Walk at a comfortable pace. If you normally use a cane or walker, be sure to do so. You can follow the program as outlined or repeat levels for a week or longer, as needed.

WEEK	SESSIONS PER WEEK	DAILY MINUTES OF WALKING	TOTAL WEEKLY MINUTES
1	2	5	10
2	3	5	15
3	4	5	20
4	5	5	25
5	5	10	50
6	5	20	100
7	5	25	125
8	5	30	150

If you're already exercising: Start at the level that best matches your current routine and build from there. Aim to walk at a moderate to brisk pace (see the definitions below). If the plan seems too easy, you may increase walking time more quickly than outlined here.

Once you've reached the goal of 150 minutes per week, feel free to vary the days and times, while maintaining the total. If it helps, you can divide daily walking time into 10-minute chunks (three chunks equals 30 minutes).

If you're looking for more of a challenge: Pick up your speed, or add time, distance, or hills to your walk to improve your endurance.

Step by step

1. Walk slowly for several minutes to warm up.

2. After that, aim for your recommended walking pace. At a light-to-moderate clip, you should be able to talk and breathe easily. Another way to gauge your pace is to count steps per minute with a watch and pedometer. Provided you're walking on level ground, you can use this guide to determine your pace:

- Slow = 80 steps per minute
- Moderate = 100 steps per minute
- Brisk = 120 steps per minute
- Fast = more than 130 steps per minute.

3. After your walk, your muscles will be nicely warmed up. This is a good time to do a balance workout or stretches.

Using the workouts

In this chapter, you'll find a list of equipment that you'll need for our workouts, explanations of terms used in the workouts, and some advice on structuring your program. Importantly, you will also find a list of both standing and seated warm-ups. Every workout should begin with a warm-up and finish with stretches (see page 47).

Choosing the right equipment

The introduction to each workout description says what equipment you'll need. Four of the six workouts require no more than a sturdy chair. The notable exception is the Balance on the Beam Workout (page 39). (When equipment is listed as optional, that means it's for an easier or harder variation of certain exercises.)

Airex Balance Beam ($130–$200) or similar product. This is a five-foot-long balance beam made of lightweight, high-density foam that sits directly on the floor. Only 2.5 inches high and 4.5 inches wide, it stores easily in a closet or under a bed. The padded, elevated surface of the beam introduces several elements that make balance exercises more challenging. If you don't have a balance beam, you can put a strip of masking tape on your floor as an alternative. However, since the surface of the floor is stable, this reduces the challenge of the workout.

Chair. Choose a sturdy chair that won't tip over easily. Unless otherwise noted in the workout description, a plain wooden dining chair without arms or heavy padding works well.

Mat. Use a well-padded nonslip mat for floor exercises. Yoga mats are readily available. A thick carpet or towels will do in a pinch.

Shoes. Select a comfortably fitted, rubber-soled shoe with little or no heel for balance exercises. One example is sneakers designed for walking. Walking shoes need to be replaced regularly because they lose support and cushioning over time. Some experts suggest buying new ones every 350 to 550 miles because the structure inside the shoes breaks down before they look like they need to be replaced.

Yoga strap. This is an inelastic cotton or nylon strap of six feet or longer that helps you position your body properly while doing the hamstring stretch. Choose a strap with a D-ring or buckle fastener on one end. This allows you to put a loop around a foot or leg and then grasp the other end of the strap. A belt or bathrobe sash will work, if you don't have a strap.

Understanding the workout instructions

When you turn to the workout you've chosen—for instance, the Beginner Balance Workout (page 26) or the Standing Balance Workout (page 29)—you'll see that each exercise has certain information and instructions. The terms we use are defined below:

Repetitions (reps). Each rep is a single complete exercise. It's fine if you can't do all the reps at first. Focus on quality rather than quantity. Good form should always come first. Gradually increase reps as you improve.

Sets. One set is a specific number of repetitions. In our workouts, 10 reps usually add up to a single set. Typically, we suggest doing one to three sets. Resting briefly after a set gives your muscles a chance to recharge, which helps you maintain good form. However, no rest is needed after stretches or after sets of exercises in which you complete all reps on one side and then repeat the reps on the other side.

Tempo. This is the count for key movements in an exercise. A 2–2–2 tempo requires you to count to two as you perform a move, hold for two beats, then count to two as you return to the starting position. To avoid hurrying, count while watching or listening to seconds tick by on a clock. When you can no longer maintain the recommended tempo, stop that particular exercise even if you haven't finished all of the reps.

Hold. Hold tells you the number of seconds or breaths to pause while holding a pose during an exercise. Many stretches, for example, are held for 10 to 30 seconds, while many yoga poses are held for one to five breaths. While starting out at 10 seconds (or one breath) is fine, gradually extending that until you can comfortably hold the stretch for 30 seconds (or a yoga pose for five breaths) will give you better results. So, too, will practicing stretches every day rather than just a few times a week.

Starting position. This describes how to position your body before starting the exercise.

Movement. This explains how to perform one complete repetition correctly.

Tips and techniques. We offer two or three pointers to help you maintain good form and make the greatest gains from the exercise.

Make it easier. This gives you an option for making the exercise less challenging.

Make it harder. This gives you an option for making the exercise more challenging.

"Neutral" is another term you'll notice in the exercises. A neutral spine takes into account the slight natural curves of the spine—don't flex your back or arch it to overemphasize the curve of the lower back. A neutral wrist is firm and straight, not bent upward or downward.

Selecting a balance workout

Some workouts are much more challenging than others. If you're not completely steady on your feet, first master the Beginner Balance Workout (page 26). These are simple, gentle balance exercises that can be done by practically anyone. If you normally need a cane or walker to keep your balance, use it during the workout as well. Be prepared to catch yourself if you start to wobble: put your hand on a counter or the back of a sturdy chair, or position yourself in the corner of a room so that you can't sway too far without support.

You can then move on to the Standing Balance Workout (page 29) and the Yoga Balance Workout (page 32).

The more challenging workouts are the Balance in Motion Workout (page 36), the Balance on the Beam Workout (page 39), and the Advanced Yoga Balance Workout (page 43). Before you try these, build your balancing skills and confidence by mastering easier workouts.

Aim to do a full balance workout two to three times a week. To improve your balance more quickly, you can also sprinkle a few simple balance exercises—single-leg stance (page 30), heel raises (page 29), side leg lifts (page 28), tandem standing (page 29), and stand up, sit down (page 27)—throughout the course of each day. Just be sure to attend to safety, and remember to keep your core muscles engaged to enhance balance (see "Three exercises to improve core strength," page 19).

And don't forget to begin each workout with a warm-up (see below) and finish with stretches (page 47). The stretching routine can be done more often—even daily—to enhance flexibility.

Warm-ups

If you walk before a balance workout, your muscles are already warmed up. Otherwise, warm up for three to five minutes before doing exercises by choosing a few of the following standing—or, if necessary, seated—options. If that's too much, a warm shower also counts as a way to warm up muscles. Here are a few warm-up options to pick from.

Standing warm-ups

- Walk or march in place.
- Do knee lifts.
- Lift your knees as you walk.
- Do toe taps.
- Dance to a few songs on the radio.

Seated warm-ups

- Roll your shoulders forward, up, back, and down.
- Do knee lifts.
- Rotate your ankles in circles.
- Tap your toes.
- Turn your head right, then left.
- Rotate your wrists in circles.
- Rotate your trunk right, then left.
- Reach up with your right arm, then your left arm. 

EASY: Beginner Balance Workout

This workout is the perfect first step toward improving shaky balance. It can be done by people of many ages and abilities, including those who are older, frail, or recovering from illness or surgery. No equipment other than a sturdy chair or counter is necessary, making this workout excellent for home or travel. If you normally need assistance from a cane or walker to balance, you should use it during this workout.

Focus on good form, rather than worrying about how many repetitions (reps) you can complete. For instance, remember to engage (tighten) your core muscles before you start each exercise. If you find an exercise especially difficult, do fewer reps or try the easier variation. As you improve, try a harder variation. (If this workout is too easy for you, begin with the Standing Balance Workout, page 29.) Before you start, be sure to read "Starting balance workouts safely," page 20.

Equipment: Sturdy chair or counter.

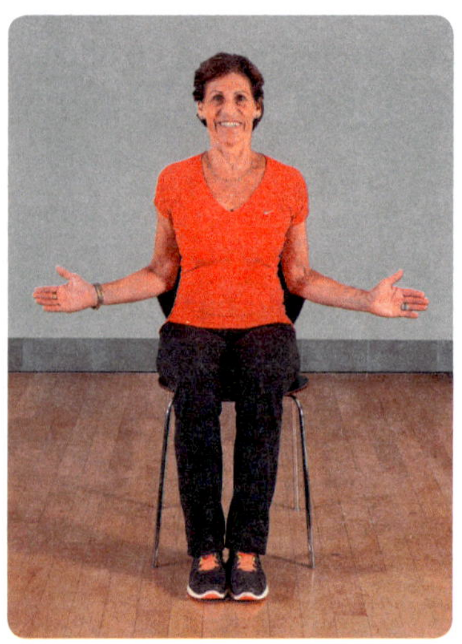

1 | Shoulder blade squeezes

Reps: 10
Sets: 1–3
Tempo: 2–4–2

Starting position: Sit up tall in a chair. Lift your chest, keeping your shoulders down and back. Tighten your abdominal muscles and bend your elbows, palms toward each other.

Movement: While exhaling, roll your shoulders farther down and back, away from your ears. Rotate your arms out so your palms face forward, squeezing your shoulder blades together. Hold. Slowly return to starting position.

Tips and techniques:

- Think of squeezing a tennis ball between your shoulder blades.
- Keep your spine neutral and tighten your abdominal muscles throughout the movement.
- Don't let your shoulders come up toward your ears; keep them down.

Make it easier: Don't rotate your arms as much; hold for only one or two counts.

Make it harder: Hold the squeeze for eight counts.

2 | Get up and go

Reps: 10
Sets: 1–3
Tempo: Go at your own pace

Starting position: Choosing a path free of obstacles, place a marker (such as a soup can or a small cone) on the floor about 10 feet from a chair. Sit in the chair with your hands on your thighs.

Movement: Stand up and walk forward to the marker. Walk around it and return to the chair. Slowly sit down in the chair. Repeat, walking in the opposite direction.

Tips and techniques:

- Keep your head and chest lifted as you stand up and sit down.
- After rising from the chair, steady yourself if necessary before walking toward the marker.
- Maintain control as you lower into the chair; don't just plop down.

Make it easier: Use a chair with armrests and use your hands to assist you as you stand up and sit down; do fewer reps.

Make it harder: Pick up your pace.

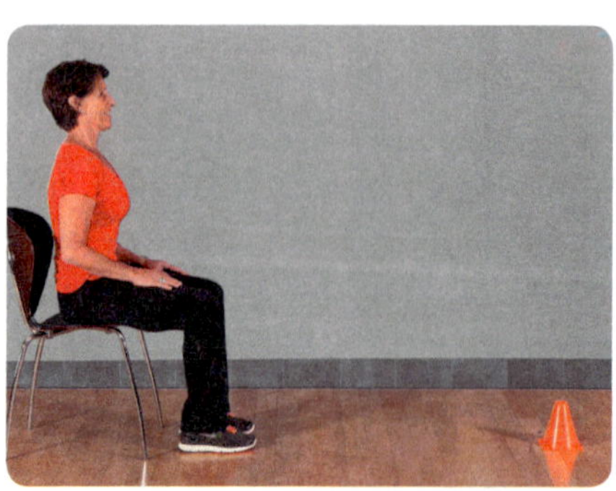

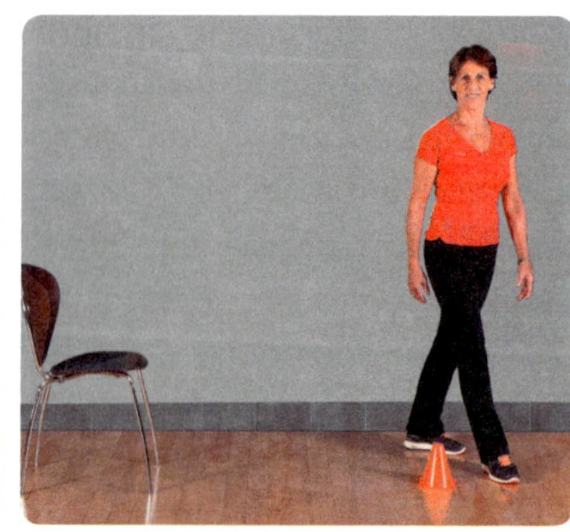

3 | Stand up, sit down

Reps: 10
Sets: 1–3
Tempo: 4–2–4

Starting position: Sit in a chair with your hands crossed on your chest or held out in front of you at chest level. Your feet should be flat on the floor, hip-width apart, and directly beneath your knees.

Movement: Lean forward slightly and slowly stand up. Hold. Slowly sit down with control.

Tips and techniques:

- Press your heels into the floor and tighten your buttocks as you stand up to help you balance.
- Steady yourself before you sit down.
- Exhale as you stand, inhale as you sit.

Make it easier: Place your hands on your thighs (or use a chair with armrests) to assist you as you stand up and sit down; do fewer reps.

Make it harder: Modify the exercise by placing your right foot slightly in front of your left one, keeping both feet flat on the floor. Stand up and sit down. Finish all reps, then repeat with the left leg in front.

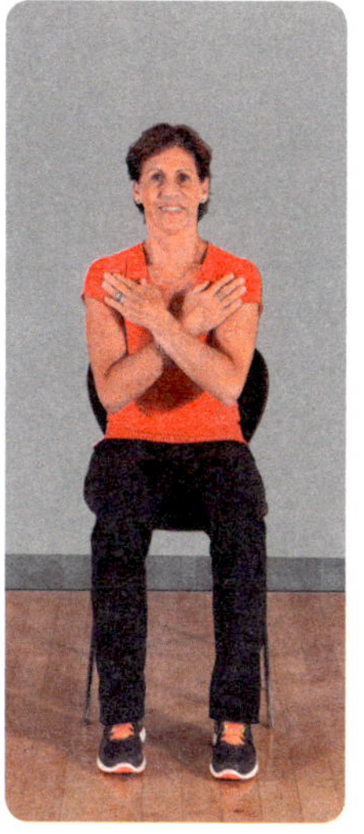

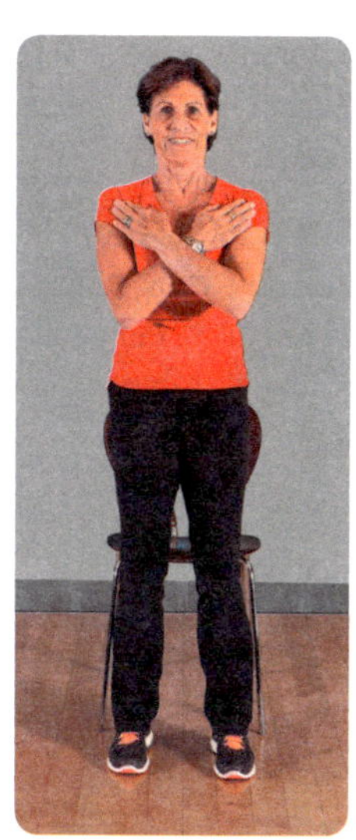

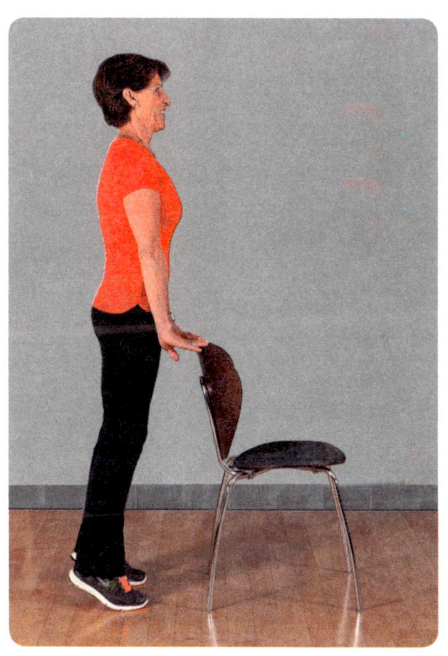

4 | Heel raises with chair support

Reps: 10
Sets: 1–3
Tempo: 2–2–2

Starting position: Stand up straight behind a chair, holding the back of it with both hands. Position your feet hip-width apart and evenly distribute your weight on both feet.

Movement: Lift your heels off the floor, shifting your weight to the balls of your feet. Try to balance evenly without allowing your ankles to roll inward or outward. Hold. Lower your heels to the floor, maintaining good posture as you do.

Tips and techniques:

- In the starting position, think of each foot as a brick and stand evenly on all four corners. When lifting, try to balance evenly on the front two corners.
- Zip your abdominal muscles up and in as if you were wearing a tight pair of jeans while tightening your buttocks and your inner thighs and balancing on the balls of your feet.
- Imagine you have a string at the top of your head pulling you up.

Make it easier: Sit down in a chair. Lift your heels off the floor. Hold. Lower your heels to the floor.

Make it harder: While holding on to the back of a chair, bend your left knee slightly to lift your foot a few inches off the floor. Do heel lifts with your right foot. Finish all reps, then repeat with your left foot.

5 | Standing side leg lift

Reps: 10 on each side
Sets: 1–3
Tempo: 2–2–2

Starting position: Stand up straight behind a chair, holding the back of it with both hands. Put your feet together and evenly distribute your weight on both feet.

Movement: Slowly lift your right leg straight out to the side about six inches off the floor. Hold. Return to starting position. Finish all reps, then repeat with the left leg. This completes one set.

Tips and techniques:

- Keep your shoulders and hips aligned throughout the exercise; don't lean to the side.
- Lift directly out to the side, not forward or back on a diagonal.
- Don't rotate your leg as you lift, but keep your knee facing forward.
- Point your foot as you lift.

Make it easier: Just touch your foot out to the side on the floor.

Make it harder: Hold your leg up for four to eight counts; close your eyes.

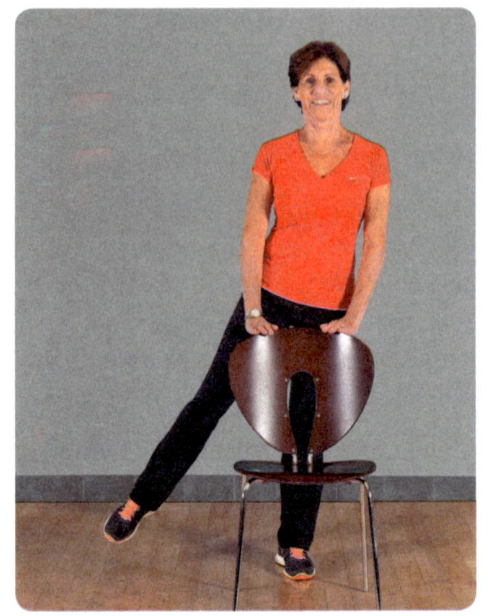

6 | Standing hamstring curls

Reps: 10 on each side
Sets: 1–3
Tempo: 2–2–2

Starting position: Stand up straight behind a chair, holding the back of it with both hands. Keeping both legs straight, extend your right leg behind you with your toes touching the floor.

Movement: Bend your right knee and try to bring the heel toward your right buttock. Hold. Slowly lower your foot to the floor. Finish all reps, then repeat with the left leg. This completes one set.

Tips and techniques:

- Maintain good posture throughout.
- Keep your hips even, tightening the buttock of the standing leg to help you balance.

Make it easier: Lift your leg less; do fewer reps.

Make it harder: Close your eyes.

▶ **You're not done yet.** See "Finish with stretches," page 47, for a set of seven stretches to end your routine. Stretching helps to prevent stiffness and preserve flexibility and range of motion.

EASY: Standing Balance Workout

Another good entry point to balance training, this workout buffs up static balance—that is, the ability to stand in one spot without swaying. If necessary, you can do many of the exercises while holding on to the back of a chair or counter for support, or standing in the corner of a room so that you can touch a wall to steady yourself.

Focus on good form, rather than worrying about how many reps you can complete. For instance, remember to engage (tighten) your core muscles before you start each exercise. If you find an exercise especially difficult, do fewer reps or try the easier variation. As you improve, try a harder variation. Before you start, be sure to read "Starting balance workouts safely," page 20.

Equipment: Sturdy chair (optional), counter (optional).

1 | Heel raises

Reps: 10
Sets: 1–3
Tempo: 2–2–2

Starting position: Stand up straight, feet hip-width apart and weight distributed evenly on both feet. Put your arms at your sides.

Movement: Lift your heels, shifting your weight to the balls of your feet. Try to balance evenly without allowing your ankles to roll inward or outward. Hold. Lower your heels to the floor, maintaining good posture as you do.

Tips and techniques:

- In the starting position, think of each foot as a brick and stand evenly on all four corners. When lifting, try to balance evenly on the front two corners.
- Zip your abdominal muscles up and in as if you were wearing a tight pair of jeans and tighten your buttocks as you stand on the balls of your feet.
- Imagine you have a string at the top of your head pulling you up.

Make it easier: Hold on to the back of a chair or a counter.

Make it harder: Hold for four to eight counts; close your eyes.

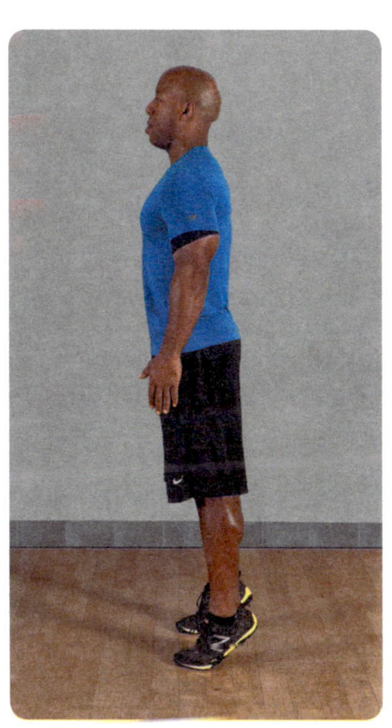

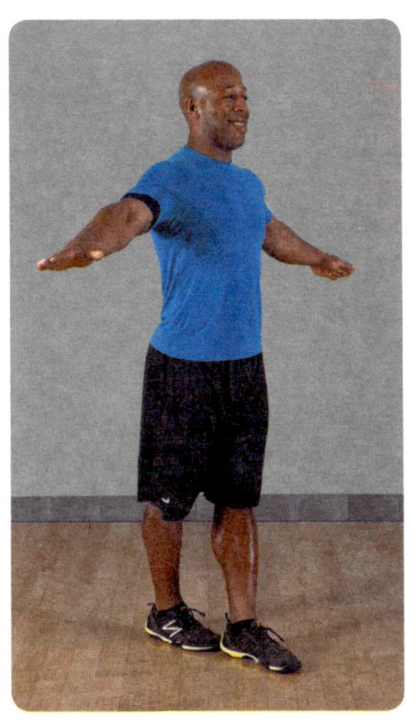

2 | Tandem standing

Reps: 1
Sets: 1–3
Hold: 5–30 seconds

Starting position: Stand up straight, feet hip-width apart and weight distributed evenly on both feet. Put your arms at your sides and engage your abdominal muscles.

Movement: Place your left foot directly in front of your right foot, heel to toe, and squeeze your inner thighs together. Lift your arms out to your sides to help you balance. Hold. Return to the starting position, then repeat with your right foot in front. This completes one rep.

Tips and techniques:

- Pick a spot straight ahead of you to focus on.
- Tighten your abdominal muscles, buttocks, and inner thighs to assist with balance.
- Keep your shoulders down and back.

Make it easier: Hold on to the back of a chair or counter with one hand.

Make it harder: Hold for 60 seconds; close your eyes.

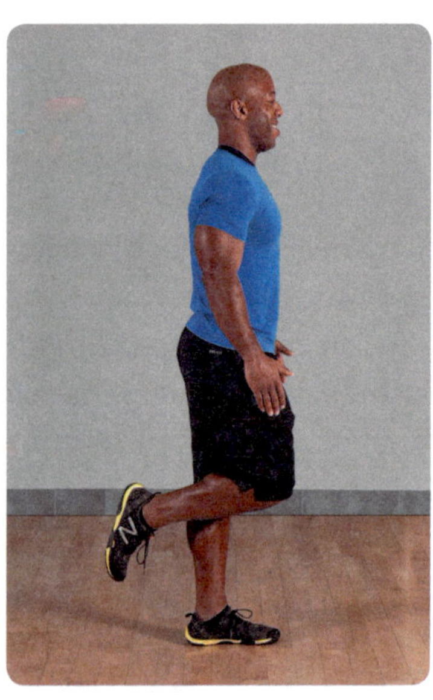

3 | Single-leg stance

Reps: 1
Sets: 1–3
Hold: 5–30 seconds

Starting position: Stand up straight, feet together and weight evenly distributed on both feet. Relax your arms at your sides.

Movement: Bend your right knee, lifting that foot several inches off the floor, and balance on your left leg. Hold. Lower your foot to the starting position, then repeat balancing on your right leg. This completes one rep.

Tips and techniques:

- Pick a spot straight ahead to focus on.
- Maintain good posture throughout by keeping your chest lifted, your shoulders down and back, and your abdominal muscles tight.
- Extend your arms out to the sides if you are wobbly.

Make it easier: Hold on to a chair or counter for support.

Make it harder: Hold for 60 seconds; close your eyes.

4 | Single-leg stance with side leg lift

Reps: 1
Sets: 1–3
Hold: 5–30 seconds

Starting position: Stand up straight, feet together and weight evenly distributed on both feet. Relax your arms at your sides.

Movement: Lift your right foot out to the side a few inches off the floor, shifting your weight over to your left leg. Lift your arms out to each side at shoulder level to help you balance. Hold. Return to the starting position, then repeat with your left foot. This completes one rep.

Tips and techniques:

- Maintain good posture throughout by keeping your chest lifted, your shoulders down and back, and your abdominal muscles tight.
- Tighten the buttock of the standing leg to help you balance.
- Keep your toes and knees pointing forward.

Make it easier: Hold on to the back of a chair or counter with one hand.

Make it harder: Hold for 60 seconds; close your eyes.

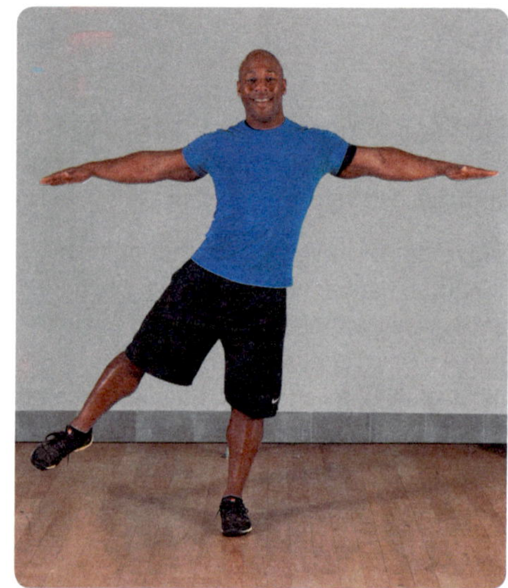

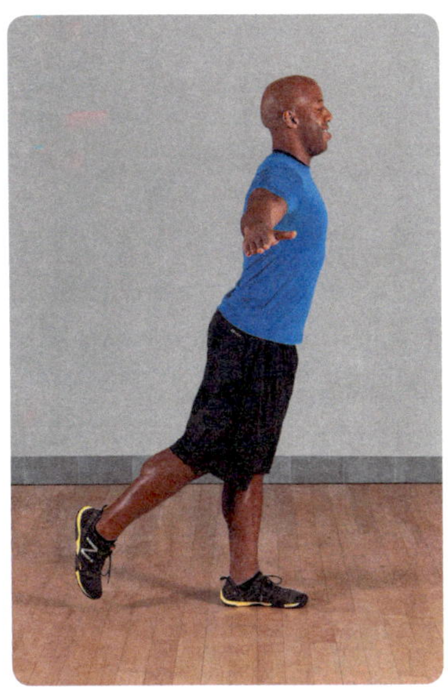

5 | Single-leg stance with back leg lift

Reps: 1
Sets: 1–3
Hold: 5–30 seconds

Starting position: Stand up straight, feet together and weight evenly distributed on both feet. Relax your arms at your sides.

Movement: Lift your right foot straight behind you a few inches off the floor, shifting your weight over to your supporting leg. Lift your arms out to your sides at shoulder level to help you balance. Hold. Return to the starting position, then repeat with your left foot. This completes one rep.

Tips and techniques:

- Pick a spot straight ahead to focus on.
- Maintain good posture throughout by keeping your chest lifted, your shoulders down and back, and your abdominal muscles tight.
- Don't lean forward more than necessary as you lift your leg. A slight forward lean is fine, but if you're leaning more than 5° to 10°, you're lifting your leg too high.

Make it easier: Hold on to the back of a chair or counter with one hand.

Make it harder: Hold for 60 seconds; close your eyes.

6 | Single-leg stance with ankle circles

Reps: 1
Sets: 1–3
Tempo: Go at your own pace

Starting position: Stand up straight with your feet together, arms at your sides, and weight evenly distributed on both feet.

Movement: Bend your right knee, lifting that leg up in front of you. Put both hands beneath the right thigh as you shift your weight over to the supporting leg. Slowly perform ankle circles with the raised foot 10 times in each direction, imagining that your toes are hitting all of the numbers on a clock face as you rotate your foot. Return to the starting position, then repeat with your left leg. This completes one rep.

Tips and techniques:

- Pick a spot straight ahead to focus on.
- Stand up straight; don't round your shoulders or hunch over.
- Tighten the buttock of the standing leg to help you balance.

Make it easier: Stand with your back against a wall, place one hand on a counter or wall for support, or sit in a chair to do the exercise.

Make it harder: Hold the single-leg stance for 60 seconds while doing ankle circles.

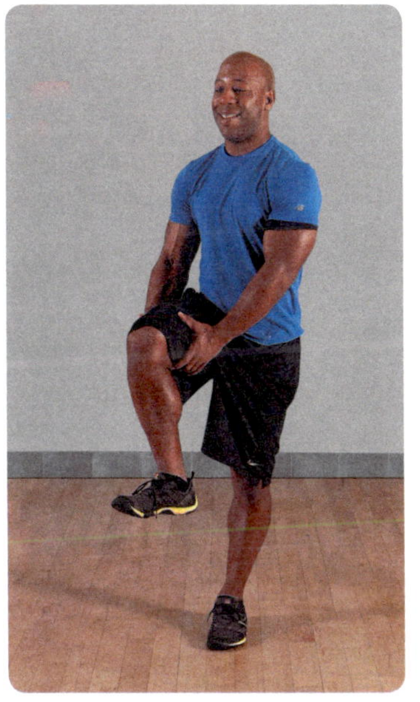

▶ **You're not done yet.** See "Finish with stretches," page 47, for a set of seven stretches to end your routine. Stretching helps to prevent stiffness and preserve flexibility and range of motion.

EASY: Yoga Balance Workout

Yoga does an excellent job of strengthening and stretching muscles essential for balance. This seven-part routine offers moves that will improve your balance, build strength, and increase flexibility while offering modifications for all levels of ability. Practice it solo for a quick yoga session; once you can do these poses without trouble, you can combine this with the Advanced Yoga Balance Workout (page 43) for a longer workout. You may also want to try yoga classes in a live group setting. That way, the instructor can help you modify the poses, if needed.

Before you start, be sure to read "Starting balance workouts safely," page 20.

Equipment: Sturdy chair.

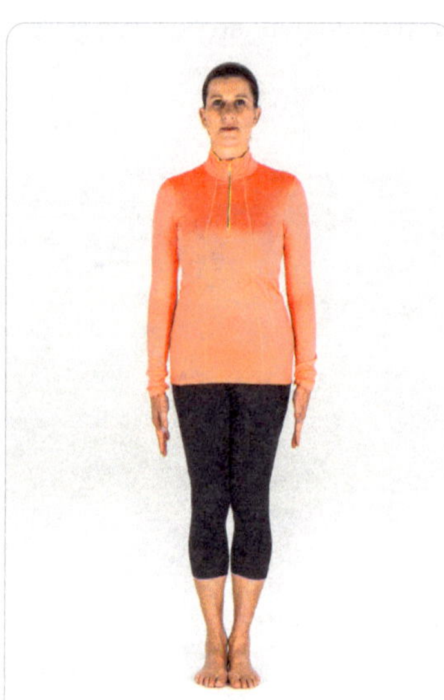

1 | Mountain pose

Reps: 1
Sets: 1
Hold: 5–10 breaths

Starting position: Stand tall with your feet together and touching. Relax your arms at your sides with your shoulders back and down.

Movement: There is no actual movement in this pose, but your body is active. Imagine your feet are firmly planted on the ground, and draw your fingertips down toward the ground. At the same time, draw your head toward the ceiling, elongating your body.

Tips and techniques:

- Don't arch or round your back.
- Don't hold your breath.
- Tighten your abdominal muscles to support your back.

2 | Tree pose

Reps: 1
Sets: 1
Hold: 5–10 breaths

Starting position: Stand tall with your feet together and touching. Relax your arms at your sides with your shoulders back and down.

Movement: As you inhale, raise your left heel off the floor, so only your left toes are touching it, and turn your leg outward. Bring your palms together in front of your chest. Hold. Release on an exhale. Repeat on the opposite leg.

Tips and techniques:

- Don't arch or round your back.
- Don't hold your breath.
- Keep your shoulders relaxed and down, away from your ears.
- Tighten your abdominal muscles to support your back.

Make it harder: Balance on one foot, placing your opposite foot on the calf of your standing leg. You can also increase the challenge by extending your arms overhead, either keeping your hands together or spreading them apart, whichever is more comfortable.

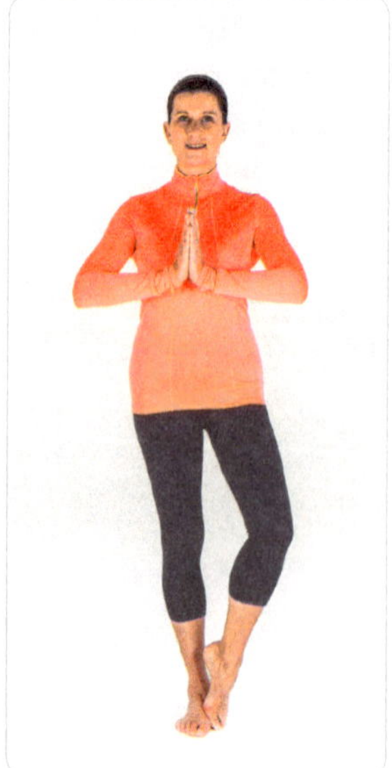

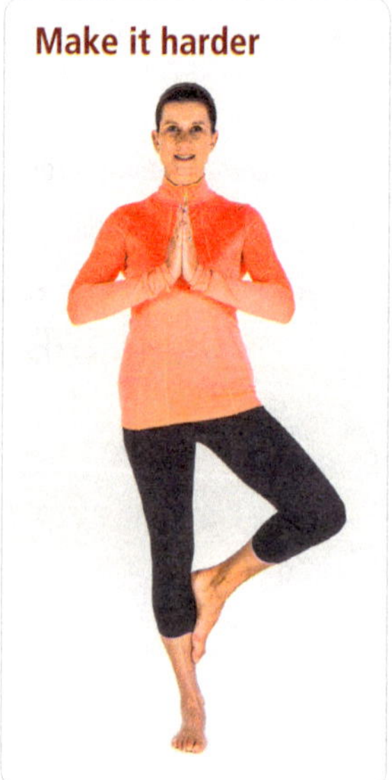

Make it harder

3 | Back bend

Reps: 3–5
Sets: 1
Hold: 3–5 breaths

Starting position: Stand up straight with your feet slightly apart. Place your hands on your lower back with your fingertips pointing down.

Movement: As you inhale, roll your shoulders back and gently lift your chest toward the ceiling, arching your back. You should be gazing up at the ceiling in front of you. Hold. Release on an exhalation.

Tips and techniques:

- Keep your shoulders relaxed and down, away from your ears.
- Don't excessively arch your back.
- Don't hyperextend your neck by looking directly above you.
- Tighten your abdominal muscles to support your back.

Make it harder: Raise your arms overhead as you arch your back.

If you have back problems or recently had abdominal surgery, check with your doctor before doing this move.

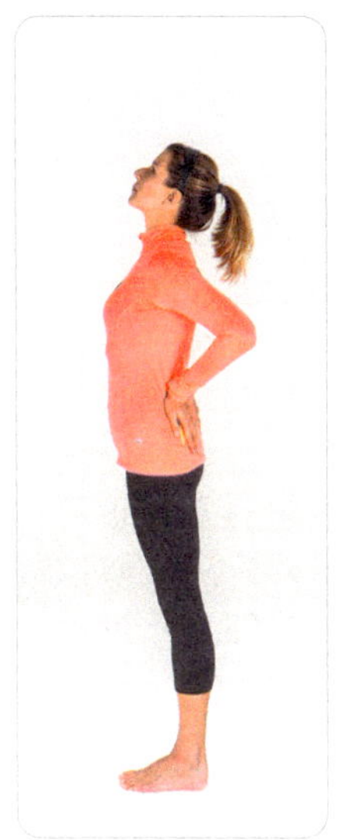

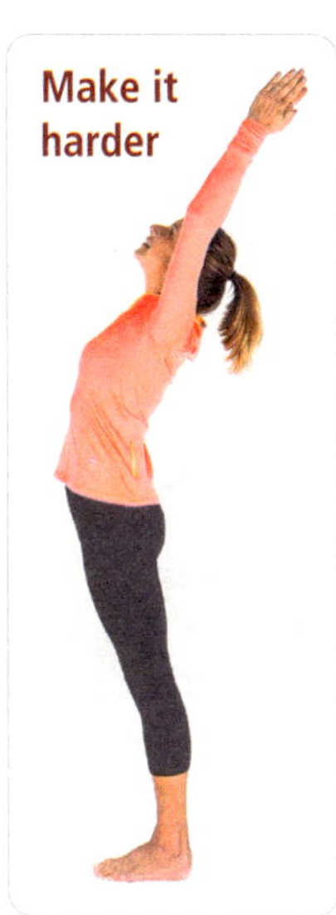

Make it harder

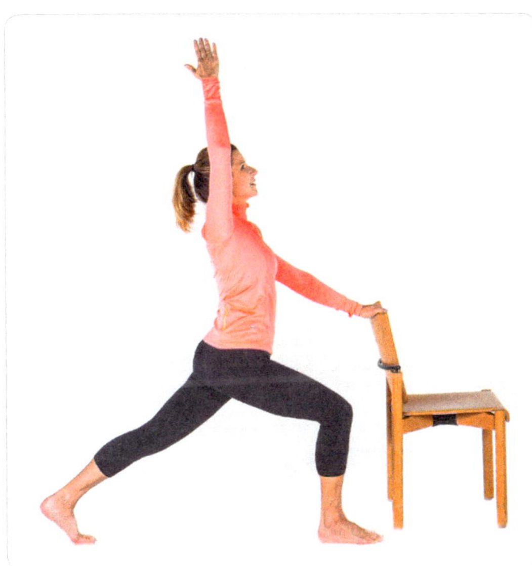

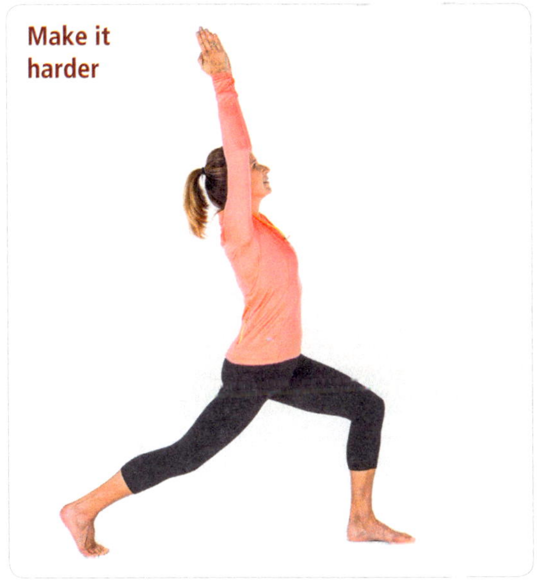

Make it harder

4 | Crescent lunge

Reps: 3–5
Sets: 1
Hold: 3–5 breaths

Starting position: Stand tall behind a chair with your feet apart slightly. Place your left hand on the back of the chair and relax your right arm at your side.

Movement: As you inhale, step back with your left foot, with your heel off the floor. Bend your right knee, lowering into a lunge and raising your right arm overhead. Hold. Inhale as you bring your feet together and exhale as you lower your arm. Repeat on the opposite side. This completes one rep.

Tips and techniques:

- Keep the movement slow and controlled.
- Keep your front knee over your ankle.
- Keep your toes pointed straight ahead.
- Tighten your abdominal muscles to support your back.

Make it harder: As you become stronger and more flexible, you can try the crescent lunge without a chair, raising both arms overhead.

5 | Forward bend

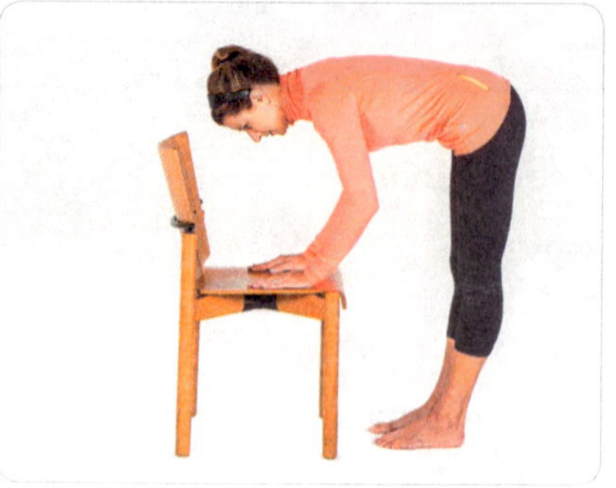

Reps: 3–5
Sets: 1
Hold: 3–5 breaths

Starting position: Stand tall in front of a chair with your feet apart slightly. Relax your arms at your sides with your shoulders back and down.

Movement: As you inhale, raise your arms overhead. As you exhale, fold forward from your hips, bringing your hands to the seat of the chair. Keep your back straight. Hold. Inhale as you stand back up, bringing your arms overhead. Exhale as you lower your arms.

Tips and techniques:

- Keep the movement slow and controlled.
- Keep your shoulders relaxed and down, away from your ears.
- Move within a comfortable range of motion. Do not strain or force any position.
- Tighten your abdominal muscles to support your back.

Make it harder: As you become more flexible, you'll be able to place your forearms on the seat of the chair. For a greater challenge, you can try the forward bend without a chair, placing your hands on your legs for support.

If you have back problems or osteoporosis, check with your doctor before doing this move.

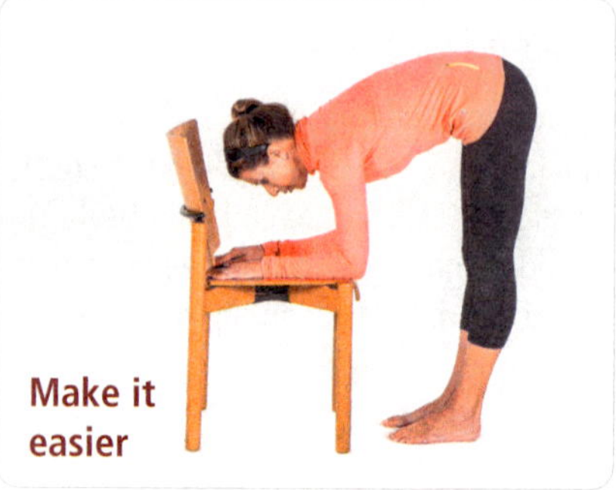
Make it easier

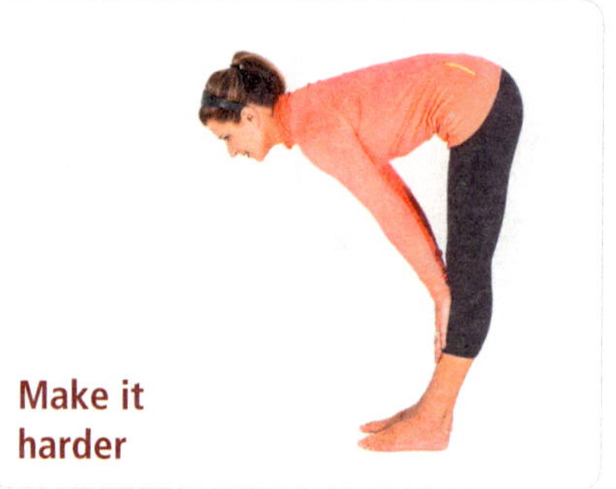
Make it harder

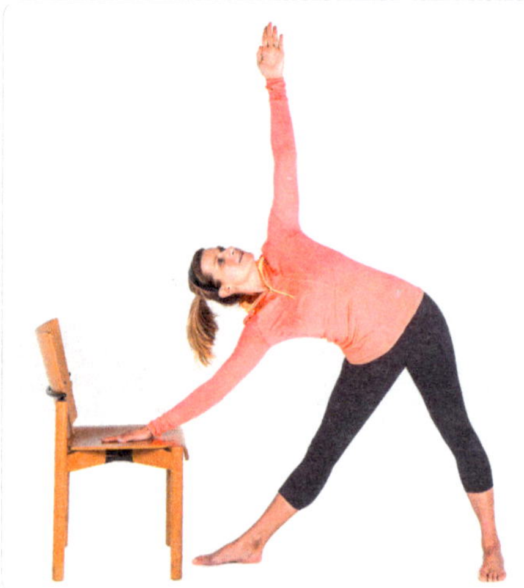

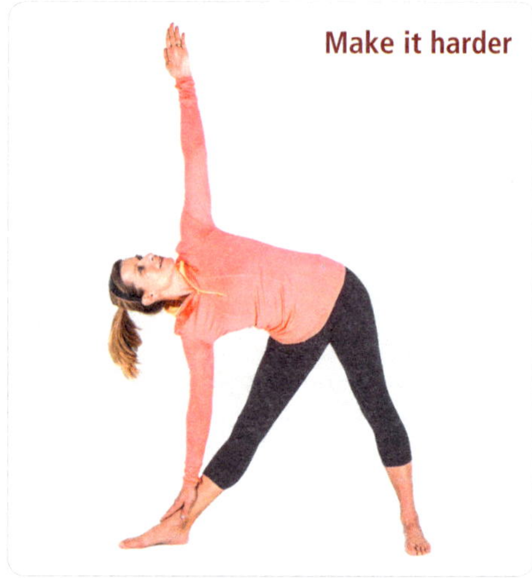
Make it harder

6 | Triangle pose

Reps: 3–5
Sets: 1
Hold: 3–5 breaths

Starting position: Stand tall with a chair to your right and spread your legs wide. Relax your arms down at your sides. Turn your right foot so it points out to the side (toward the chair), while keeping your left foot pointing forward. Your hips and shoulders should also be facing forward.

Movement: As you inhale, raise your arms to shoulder height. As you exhale, stretch your right arm and torso to the right as far as possible, then bend to the right and place your right hand on the chair seat. Raise your left arm toward the ceiling and look up at it. Hold. Stretch your fingertips toward the ceiling. Inhale as you come up, and exhale as you lower your arms. Repeat on the opposite side. This completes one rep.

Tips and techniques:

- Don't let your top hip or shoulder roll forward.
- Tighten your abdominal muscles to support your back.
- Place your hand on your hip if holding your arm up becomes tiring.

Make it harder: As you become stronger, you can try triangle pose without a chair, placing your hand on your leg wherever comfortable.

7 | Warrior II

Reps: 3–5
Sets: 1
Hold: 3–5 breaths

Starting position: Stand tall in front of a chair and spread your legs wide. Relax your arms down at your sides. Turn your right foot so it points out to the side and angle your left foot forward. Keep your hips and shoulders facing front.

Movement: As you inhale, raise your arms to shoulder height. As you exhale, bend your right knee, lowering onto the chair in a lunge position. Hold. Inhale as you straighten your legs, rising up, and exhale as you lower your arms. Repeat on the opposite side. This completes one rep.

Tips and techniques:

- Keep your front knee over your ankle.
- Reach with your fingertips toward opposite walls.
- Tighten your abdominal muscles to support your back.
- Place your hands on your hips if holding your arms up becomes tiring.

Make it harder: As you become stronger, try Warrior II without a chair.

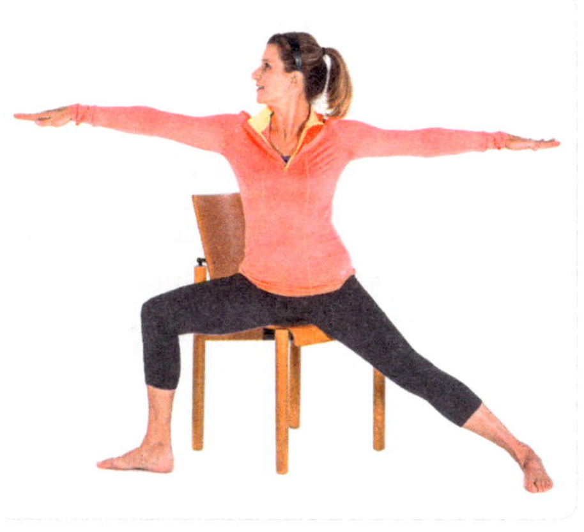

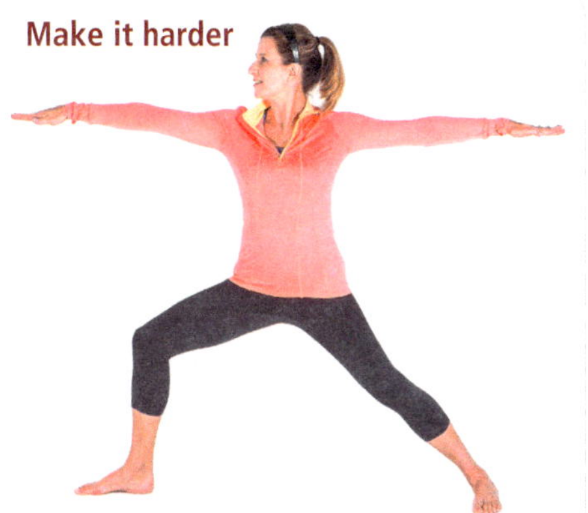

Make it harder

▶ **You're not done yet.** See "Finish with stretches," page 47, for a set of seven stretches to end your routine. Stretching helps to prevent stiffness and preserve flexibility and range of motion.

HARD: Balance in Motion Workout

Everyday acts—strolling down the street, walking up or down stairs, turning to look behind you—demand dynamic balance, the ability to anticipate and react to changes as you move. This workout hones that ability considerably, which helps prevent falls.

If you've had a hip replacement, ask your doctor if you need to modify any of the movements, particularly in exercise 2 (braiding). Otherwise, focus on good form, rather than worrying about how many reps you can complete. For instance, remember to engage (tighten) your core muscles before you start each exercise. If you find an exercise especially difficult, do fewer reps or try the easier variation. As you improve, try a harder variation. Before you start, be sure to read "Starting balance workouts safely," page 20.

Equipment: Sturdy chair (optional).

1 | Soccer kick

Reps: 10 on each side
Sets: 1–3
Tempo: 2–1–2

Starting position: Stand up straight with your feet together and your hands on your hips.

Movement: Point your right foot out to the right side and lift your arms out to the sides at shoulder level. Lift up your right foot and slowly sweep it diagonally in front of you as if kicking a soccer ball with the inside of your foot. Hold. Slowly bring your foot back to the right side. Finish all reps, then repeat with the left leg. This completes one set.

Tips and techniques:

- Keep your hips even and facing forward, and maintain neutral posture throughout.
- Tighten your abdominal muscles and the buttock of the standing leg.
- Don't rotate your upper body.

Make it easier: Hold on to the back of a chair with one hand for support.

Make it harder: Hold for four counts; don't touch your foot to the floor between reps.

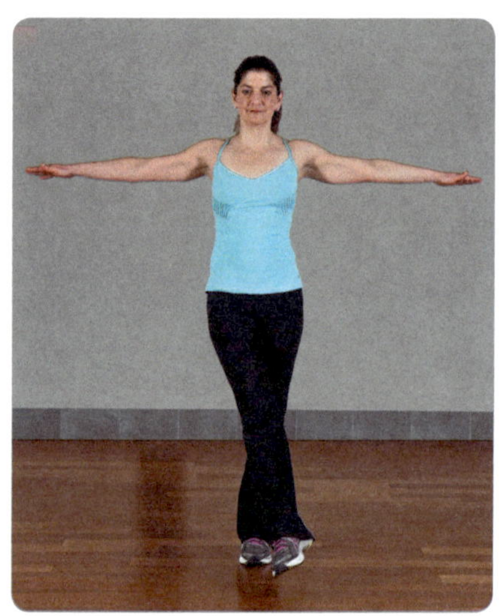

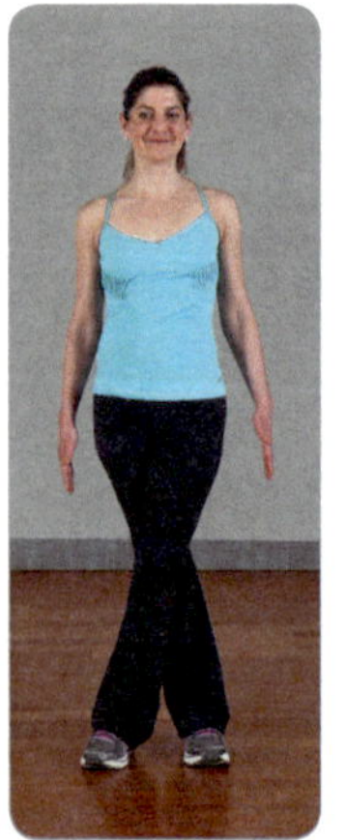

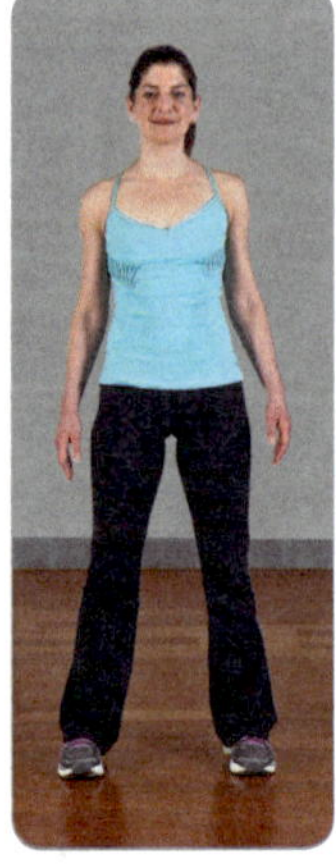

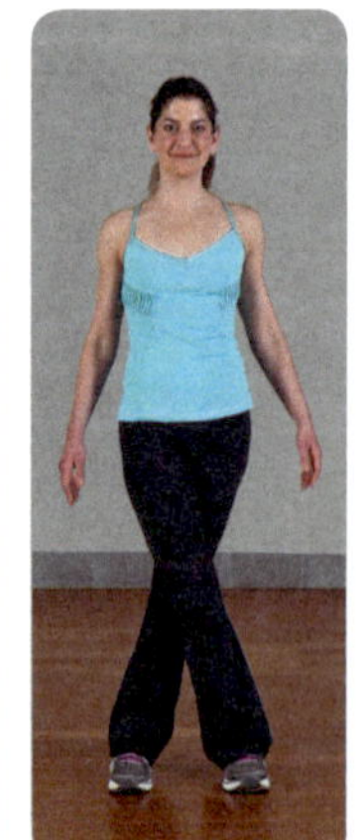

2 | Braiding

Reps: 10 to each side
Sets: 1–3
Tempo: Slow and controlled

Starting position: Stand up straight, feet together and weight evenly distributed on both feet. Put your arms at your sides.

Movement: Step toward the right with your right foot. Cross in front with your left foot, step out again with the right foot, and cross behind with your left foot. Continue this braiding for 10 steps to the right, alternating stepping in front of and behind your right foot, then bring your feet together. Hold until steady. Now do 10 steps of braiding to the left side of the room. This completes one set.

Tips and techniques:

- Maintain neutral posture throughout.
- Look ahead of you instead of down at your feet.
- Don't turn your feet out.

Make it easier: Take smaller steps.

Make it harder: Pick up your pace while staying in control of the movement.

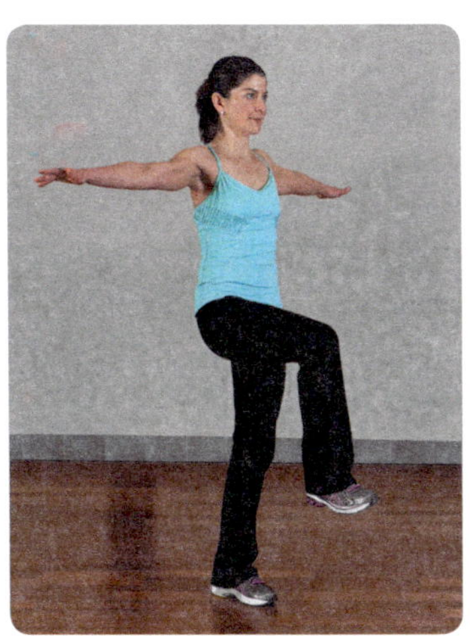

3 | Rock step

Reps: 10 on each side
Sets: 1–3
Tempo: 2–2–2–2

Starting position: Stand up straight, feet together and weight evenly distributed on both feet. Lift your arms out to each side.

Movement: Step forward with your left foot and lift up your right knee. Hold. Step back with your right foot and lift up your left knee. This completes one rep. Finish all reps with the left foot leading, then repeat with the right foot leading. This completes one set.

Tips and techniques:

- Tighten the buttock of the standing leg for stability.
- Maintain good posture throughout.
- Breathe comfortably.

Make it easier: Hold on to the back of a chair with one hand for support; lift your knee less.

Make it harder: Hold each knee up for a count of four.

4 | Side squat with knee lift and rotation

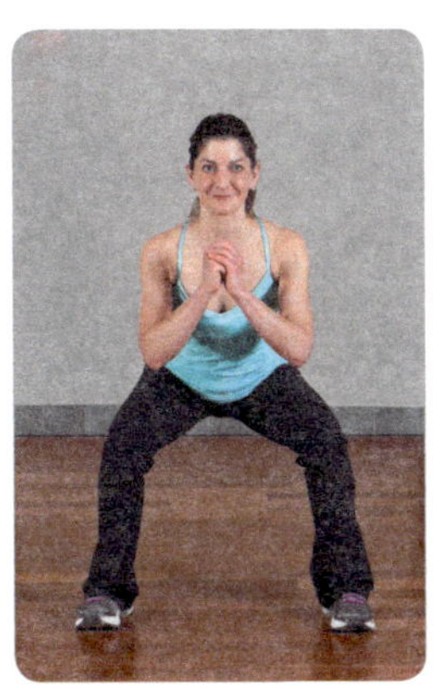

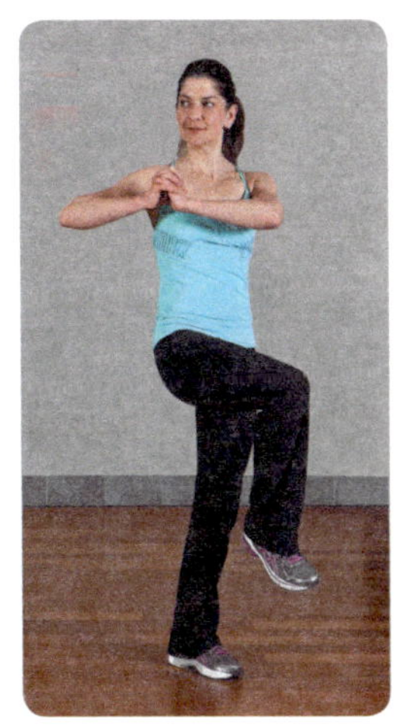

Reps: 10 on each side
Sets: 1–3
Tempo: 2–2

Starting position: Stand up straight with your feet together and your arms at your sides.

Movement: Step out to the right, hinge at your hips, and bend your knees to lower your buttocks into a squat as if sitting in a chair. Simultaneously, clasp your hands loosely in front of your chest. As you stand back up, raise your right knee while rotating your upper body to the right. Return to the squat. This is one rep. Finish all reps, then repeat the sequence stepping out to the left. This completes one set.

Tips and techniques:

- Keep your spine neutral and your shoulders down and back.
- Extend your knees no farther forward than your toes (if you look down you should be able to see your toes) and keep them pointing forward as you squat.
- Hinge your upper body slightly forward, keeping your chest lifted as you squat.

Make it easier: As you stand up, lift one knee up in front of you without twisting. If this is still too challenging, simply do squats without a knee lift or rotation.

Make it harder: Hold the squat, the knee lift, or both for two to four counts.

5 | Curtsies

Reps: 10 on each side
Sets: 1–3
Tempo: 2–2

Starting position: Stand up straight with your right leg out to your side, toe touching the floor. Extend your arms to each side at shoulder level.

Movement: Bring your right foot behind your left leg, place your weight on the ball of the rear foot, and bend your knees as if curtsying. Touch your right hand to your left knee. Press with your front foot to stand up and return to the starting position. Finish all reps, then repeat with your left leg. This completes one set.

Tips and techniques:

- Keep your spine neutral and your shoulders down and back.
- Keep your upper body facing forward the entire time.
- When returning to the starting position, tighten the buttock of your front leg as you lift up to help you balance.

Make it easier: Do fewer reps; don't lower as much.

Make it harder: As you rise up from the curtsy, lift your leg out to the side in the air, then return to the curtsy without touching the floor in between.

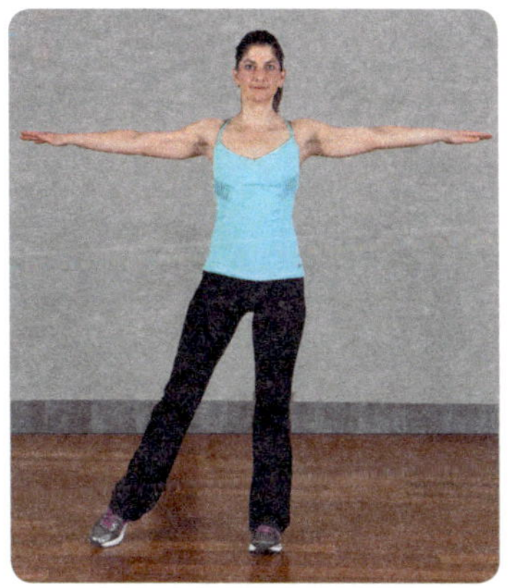

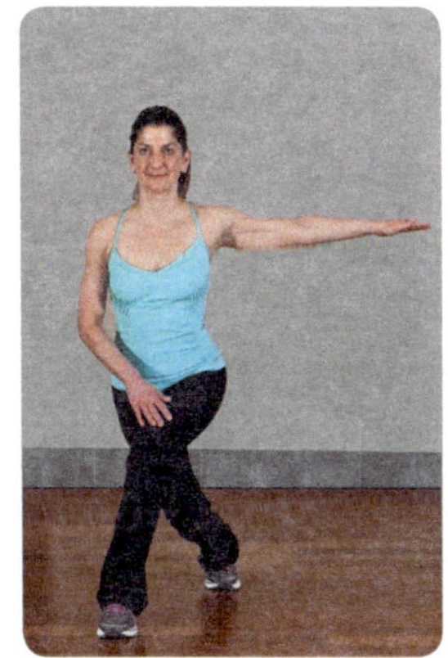

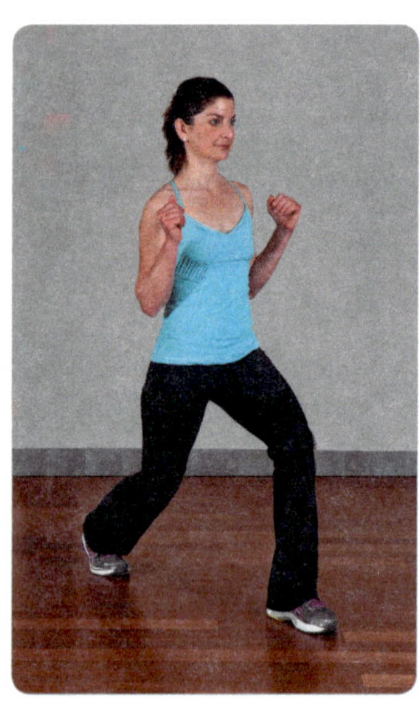

6 | Reverse lunge

Reps: 10 on each side
Sets: 1–3
Tempo: 2–2

Starting position: Stand up straight, feet together and weight evenly distributed on both feet. Relax your arms at your sides.

Movement: Step back with your right foot, landing on the ball of your right foot. Keeping your torso erect, bend both knees and lower until your left thigh is parallel to the floor. Your left knee should align with your left ankle and your right knee should point to the floor without touching it. Simultaneously, bring your hands up in front of your chest, elbows bent. Press with both feet to stand up and return to the starting position. Finish all reps, then repeat stepping back with your left foot. This completes one set.

Tips and techniques:

- Keep your front knee directly over your ankle.
- In the lunge position, your shoulder, hip, and rear knee should be aligned vertically.
- Keep your spine neutral, and don't lean forward or back.

Make it easier: Stand with one foot in front of the other and do stationary lunges, moving up and down without stepping back and forth; don't lower as much when you lunge back; do fewer reps.

Make it harder: Hold the lunge for four counts before returning to the starting position.

▶ **You're not done yet.** See "Finish with stretches," page 47, for a set of seven stretches to end your routine. Stretching helps to prevent stiffness and preserve flexibility and range of motion.

Hard: Balance on the Beam Workout

This advanced workout steps up the challenge to your balance in three ways. The soft, high-density foam surface of the Airex Balance Beam introduces instability. The raised height, though only two-and-a-half inches, puts your feet at different levels in certain exercises, much as you would encounter when stepping off a curb. In other exercises, keeping both feet on the four-and-a-half-inch-wide beam makes balancing more difficult. Mastering this workout will do a great deal to enhance your balance. Note: If you are older and have walking problems, a strip of masking tape on the floor is a safe substitute for the balance beam.

You may do this workout barefoot or wearing sneakers. Focus on good form, rather than worrying about how many reps you can complete. For instance, remember to engage (tighten) your core muscles before you start each exercise. If you find an exercise especially difficult, do fewer reps or try the variation under "Make it easier." As you improve, try the harder variation. Before you start, be sure to read "Starting balance workouts safely," page 20.

Equipment: Airex Balance Beam or similar product (see "Choosing the right equipment," page 24), or masking tape (optional).

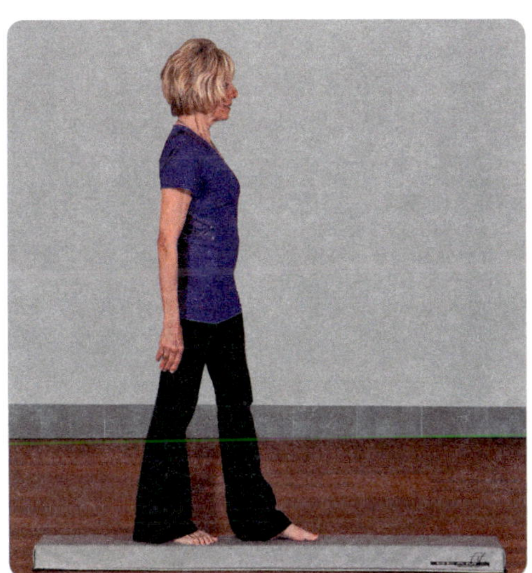

1 | Mambo step

Reps: 10 on each side
Sets: 1–3
Tempo: 2–2

Starting position: Stand up straight at the center of the balance beam. Position your left foot about four inches ahead of your right foot. Relax your arms at your sides.

Movement: During the mambo, you rock one foot forward and back. Using this mambo rhythm, slowly bring your right foot forward ahead of the left foot, press down momentarily on the beam, then slowly bring your right foot back to the starting position. As you do the step, let your arms swing comfortably slightly backward and forward as a counterbalance. Stepping forward and backward this way, finish all reps, then repeat the sequence starting with your right foot in front. This completes one set.

Tips and techniques:

- Tighten your inner thighs to help you balance.
- Pick a spot straight ahead to focus on.
- Tighten your abdominal muscles throughout the movement.

Make it easier: Do the exercise on the floor.

Make it harder: Instead of doing the mambo step, try swinging your rear foot forward and then backward in the air without touching the balance beam. Finish all reps, then repeat with the other foot.

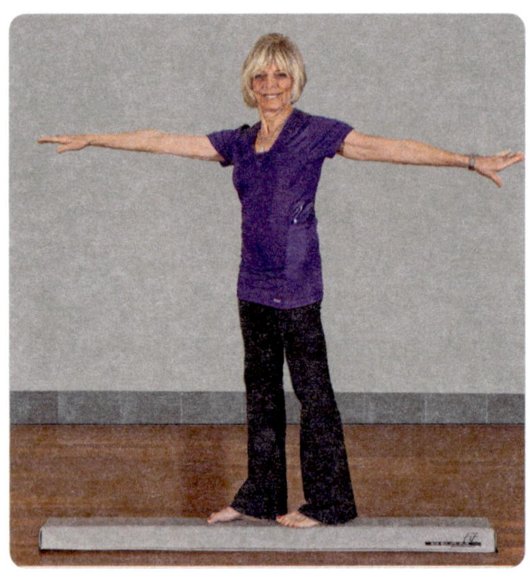

2 | Tandem stand with rotation

Reps: 5 on each side
Sets: 1–3
Tempo: 2–2–2

Starting position: Stand up straight at the center of the balance beam with your right foot positioned directly in front of your left foot, heel to toe. Relax your arms at your sides.

Movement: Bring your arms out to each side at shoulder level. Slowly rotate your head and torso toward the left side of the room. Hold. Slowly return to the starting position. Finish all reps, then repeat the sequence with your left foot forward, rotating your head and torso to the right side of the room. This completes one set.

Tips and techniques:

- Tighten your inner thighs to help you balance.
- Keep your weight evenly distributed on both feet.
- Tighten your abdominal muscles throughout the movement.

Make it easier: Do the exercise on the floor.

Make it harder: Hold the rotation for four counts.

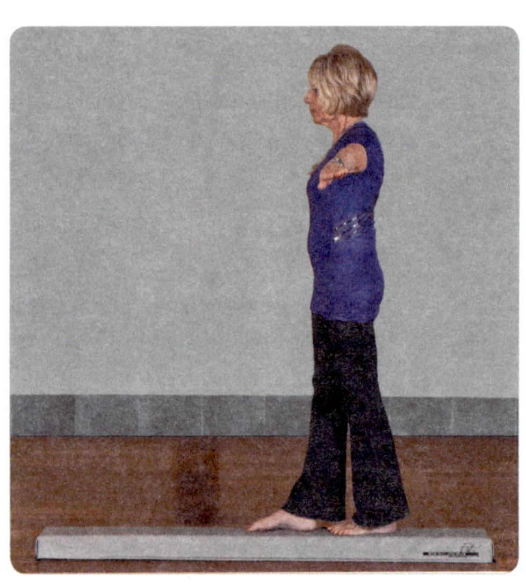

3 | Walk forward, walk back

Reps: 10 on each side
Sets: 1–3
Tempo: 2–2

Starting position: Stand up straight near one end of the balance beam. Position your right foot in front of your left foot. Relax your arms at your sides.

Movement: Lift your arms out to each side at shoulder level. Step forward several inches on the beam with your right foot, then slide your left foot forward to the heel of your right foot. Step forward again with your right foot, then slide your left foot forward. Step backward several inches on the beam with your left foot, then slide your right foot backward to the toes of your left foot. Step backward again with your left foot, then slide your right foot backward. This is one rep. Finish all reps, then repeat with your left foot forward. This completes one set.

Tips and techniques:

- Tighten your abdominal muscles throughout the movement.
- As you bring your feet together, squeeze your inner thighs together to help you balance.
- Maintain neutral posture.

Make it easier: Do the exercise on the floor.

Make it harder: Step forward, slide forward, step forward, slide forward, lift the knee of the front leg to about hip height, and then put that foot back on the beam. Step backward, slide backward, step backward, slide backward, lift the knee of the front leg to about hip height, and then put that foot back on the beam. Finish all reps, then repeat with the other leg forward.

4 | Rock step with knee lifts

Reps: 10 on each side
Sets: 1–3
Tempo: 2–2

Starting position: Stand up straight on the balance beam. Position your right foot in front of your left foot and extend your arms out to each side at shoulder level.

Movement: Slowly step forward on the beam with your right foot and lift your left knee to about hip height. Step backward onto the center of the beam behind you with your left foot and lift your right knee to about hip height. This completes one rep. Finish all reps, then repeat with your left foot forward. (The rocking motion gives this exercise its name.) This completes one set.

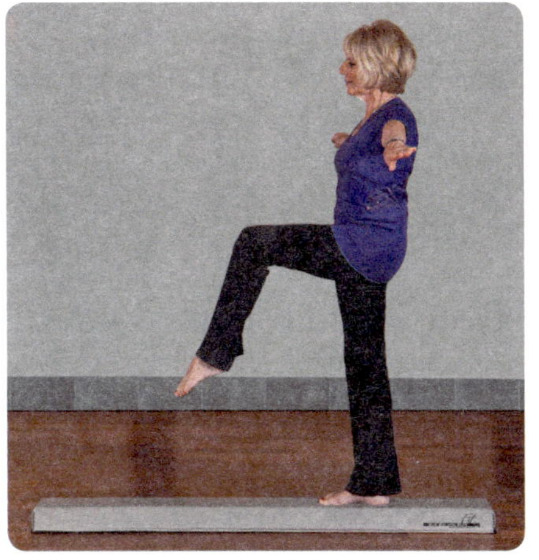

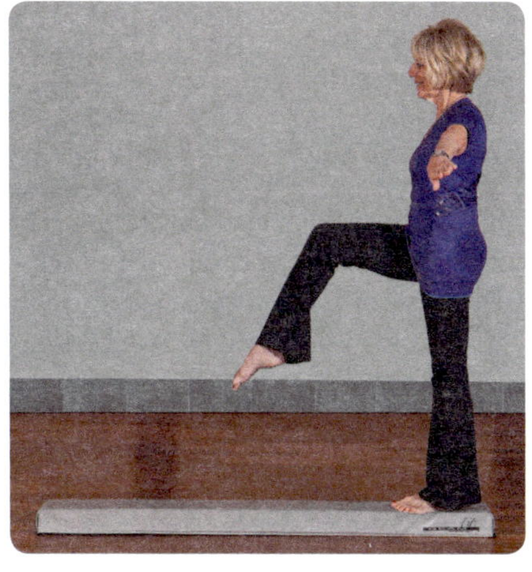

Tips and techniques:

- Maintain neutral posture.
- Always step in the center of the beam.
- Tighten your abdominal muscles and tighten the buttock of the standing leg to help you balance.

Make it easier: Do the exercise on the floor.

Make it harder: Hold the knee lifts for two counts.

5 | Stationary lunge

Reps: 10 on each side
Sets: 1–3
Tempo: 2–2

Starting position: Stand up straight with your right foot in front of your left foot, about two feet apart. Your right foot should be flat, and you should be on the ball of your left foot. Extend your arms out to your sides at shoulder level to help with balance.

Movement: Keeping your torso erect, slowly bend both knees and lower until your right thigh is parallel to the beam. Your right knee should align over your right ankle, and your left knee should point down toward the beam without touching it. Slowly straighten your legs, returning to the starting position. Finish all reps, then repeat with your left foot in front. This completes one set.

Tips and techniques:

- Keep your abdominal muscles tight throughout the movement.
- Maintain neutral posture and don't lean forward or back.
- Keep your front knee directly over your ankle.

Make it easier: Don't lower as much; do the exercise on the floor.

Make it harder: Hold the lunge for four counts.

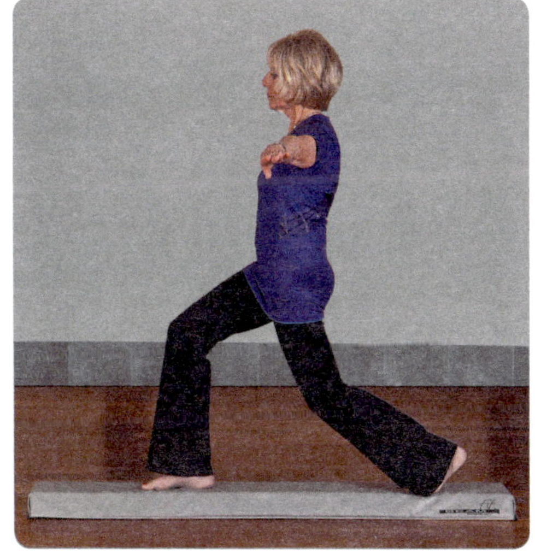

6 | Side squat, forward lunge

Reps: 10 on each side
Sets: 1–3
Tempo: 2–2–2–2

Starting position: Stand up straight at the center of the balance beam. Position your right foot a few inches ahead of your left foot and raise your arms to the side at shoulder level.

Movement: This four-part movement is side squat, forward lunge, side squat, stand. First, step to the left of the balance beam with your left foot, hinging forward at your hips and bending your knees into a squat as if sitting down in a chair, while clasping your hands loosely in front of your chest with elbows bent. Second, lift up from the squat, bring your left foot to the front of the balance beam, and sink into a small lunge by bending both knees so that the left knee aligns over your left ankle and the right knee points to the beam. Let your right arm swing forward and your left arm swing slightly backward as a counterbalance. Third, lift up from the lunge and return to the side squat position with hands clasped loosely in front of your chest. Fourth, lift up once more from the squat and bring your feet back to the starting position, your right foot a few inches ahead of your left foot, as you raise your arms out to each side at shoulder level. This completes one rep. Finish all reps, then repeat with your left foot forward so that the squat is to the right side. This completes one set.

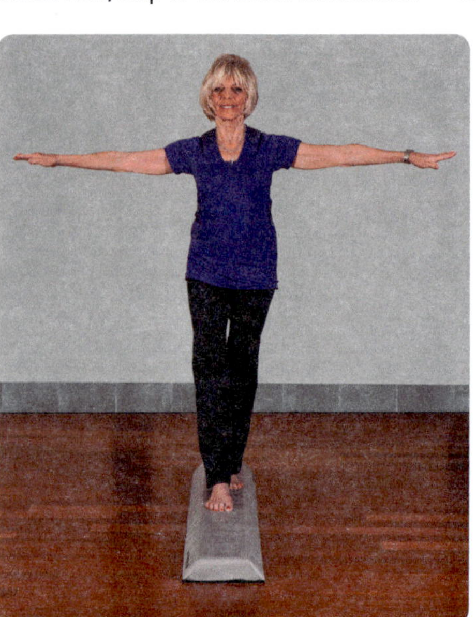

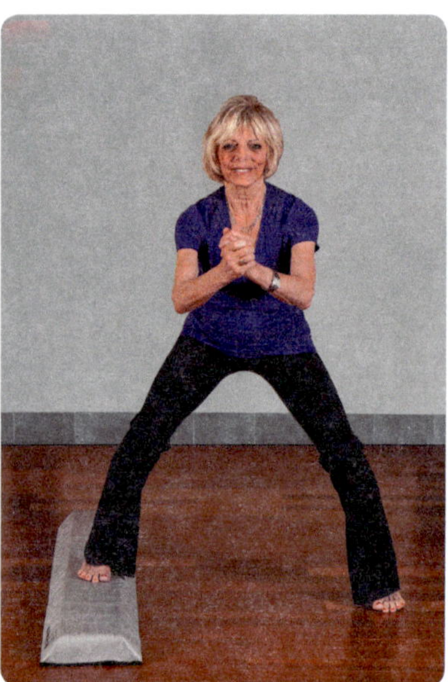

Tips and techniques:

- Tighten your abdominal muscles and maintain neutral posture throughout the movement.
- Tighten the buttock of the leg on the beam to help you balance.
- Don't let your knees extend beyond your toes when you squat.

Make it easier: Do the exercise on the floor.

Make it harder: Hold the lunge for four counts instead of two.

▶ **You're not done yet.** See "Finish with stretches," page 47, for a set of seven stretches to end your routine. Stretching helps to prevent stiffness and preserve flexibility and range of motion.

HARD: Advanced Yoga Balance Workout

These yoga poses challenge both static balance (the ability to stand in one spot without swaying) and dynamic balance (the ability to anticipate and react to changes as you move). Successfully managing these tasks requires you to keep your center of gravity poised over a base of support. Focus on good form, rather than worrying about how many reps you can complete. For instance, remember to engage your core muscles before you start each exercise. If you find an exercise especially difficult, do fewer reps or try the easier variation. As you improve, try the harder variation. Before you start, be sure to read "Starting balance workouts safely," page 20.

Equipment: Mat.

Yoga breathing

Yoga breathing, or pranayama, is relaxing and meditative. Try this simple technique while performing yoga poses, or do it for a few minutes once or twice during the day. To learn the technique, follow these steps.

1. Lie on a mat with your knees bent and feet flat on the floor, hip-width apart. Rest one hand on your heart and the other below your navel. Inhale and exhale through your nose, if possible (if not, breathe in through the nose, and out through softly parted lips). As you exhale, try to make a whispering sound at the back of your throat.

2. Start tuning in to the way you breathe. Notice how the air feels as it enters and exits your nostrils.

3. As you continue, begin counting silently (one, two, three, four) on the inhale and then on the exhale. Gradually lengthen your breaths until each exhalation is twice as long as each inhalation. As you fill your lungs, feel your rib cage expand to the side and your lower belly rise and fall slightly. Focus on breathing slowly and smoothly.

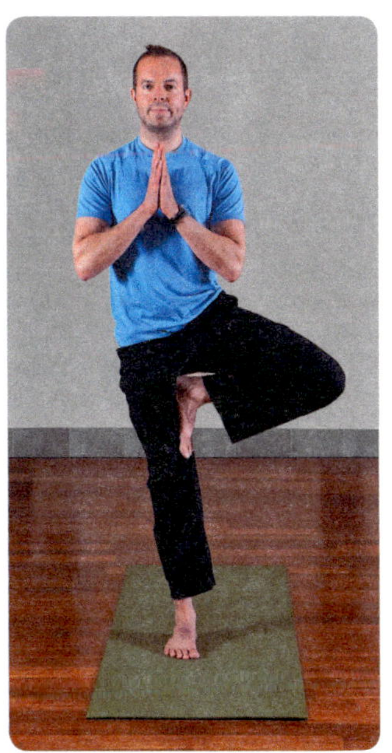

1 | Tree pose

Reps: 2–4
Sets: 1
Hold: 10 breaths

Starting position: Stand up straight, feet together and weight evenly distributed on both feet. Relax your arms at your sides.

Movement: Slowly shift your weight to your right leg. Lift up your left foot and place it on the inside of your right leg above or below the knee. To help you balance, place the sole of your left foot firmly against your right leg and press your right leg against your left foot, grounding down through the standing leg for stability. Engage your abdominal muscles as you bend your elbows and bring your hands up in front of your chest in a prayer position. Hold. Return to the starting position, then repeat standing on your left leg. This completes one rep.

Tips and techniques:

- Pick a spot straight ahead to focus on.
- Don't place your foot on your opposite knee.
- Tighten the buttock of the standing leg to help you balance.

Make it easier: Place your foot at your calf or just above the ankle of the supporting leg.

Make it harder: Lift your foot higher on the supporting leg so that the heel is near your groin.

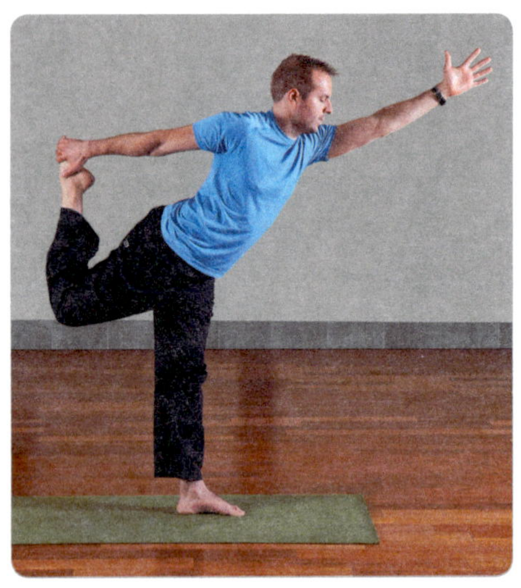

2 | Dancer

Reps: 2–4
Sets: 1
Hold: 5 breaths

Starting position: Stand up straight, feet together and weight evenly distributed on both feet. Relax your arms at your sides.

Movement: Raise your left arm forward at shoulder level, thumb up. Bend your right knee and reach back with your right hand to grasp your ankle or your foot and lift it toward your buttock. Inhale and lift your left arm higher and lean forward slightly as you raise your right leg behind you. Hold. Return to the starting position, then repeat bending your left leg. This completes one rep.

Tips and techniques:

- Pick a spot straight ahead to focus on.
- Tighten your abdominal muscles and the buttock of the standing leg.
- Don't let your back leg rotate out to the side.

Make it easier: Instead of raising your arm, hold on to a sturdy chair or put one hand against the wall.

Make it harder: Hold for 10 breaths.

3 | Crescent warrior

Reps: 2–4
Sets: 1
Hold: 5 breaths

Starting position: Stand up straight, feet together and weight evenly distributed on both feet. Relax your arms at your sides.

Movement: Place your hands on your right thigh as you step back onto the ball of your left foot and sink into a high lunge by bending your right knee so that it is aligned over the ankle. Keep your left leg straight and your head, shoulders, hips, and feet facing forward. Bring your hands out to each side at shoulder level, palms up. Slowly exhale and rotate your torso to the right as far as comfortable, keeping your chin centered above your chest. Hold. Return to the starting position, then repeat by stepping back onto the ball of your right foot and rotating your torso toward the left. This completes one rep.

Tips and techniques:

- Tighten your abdominal muscles throughout.
- Try to keep your weight evenly distributed between both feet.
- Keep your front knee from extending beyond your toes.

Make it easier: Skip the rotation.

Make it harder: Hold for 10 breaths.

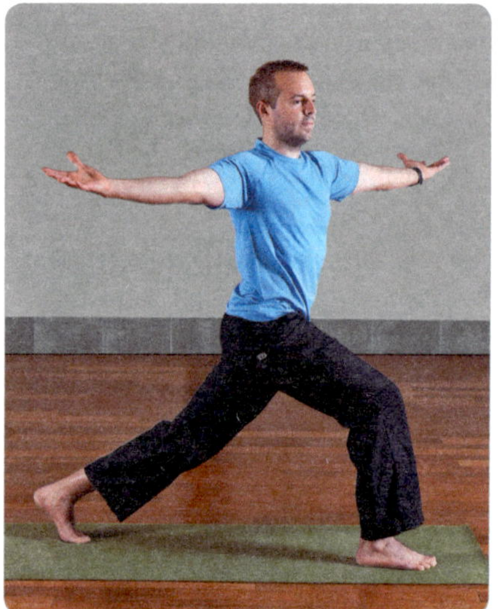

4 | Warrior III

Reps: 2–4 on each side
Sets: 1
Hold: 5 breaths

Starting position: Stand up straight, feet together and weight evenly distributed. Place your hands on your right thigh as you step back onto the ball of your left foot and sink into a high lunge by bending your right knee so that it is aligned over the ankle. Keep your left leg straight, and your head, shoulders, hips, and feet facing forward.

Movement: Shift your weight forward over your right leg. Simultaneously lift both arms forward in line with your shoulders, palms inward, and lift your left leg until it is parallel to the floor, flexing the ankle so that your toes point toward the floor. Your head, shoulders, and hips should be even and parallel to the floor. Hold. Exhale and return to the starting position. Finish all reps. Repeat the full sequence with your weight on your left leg.

Tips and techniques:

- Tighten your abdominal muscles and the buttock of the supporting leg to help you balance.
- Think of someone pulling your arms forward and drawing your extended leg backward.
- Keep your head and spine neutral and your shoulders down (away from your ears).

Make it easier: Slightly bend the knee of your supporting leg and do not lift your back leg as high.

Make it harder: As you raise your back leg, bring your arms back alongside your body, palms toward the floor.

5 | Side plank

Reps: 2–4 on each side
Sets: 1
Hold: 10 breaths

Starting position: Kneel on all fours with your hands and knees directly aligned under your shoulders and hips. Extend both legs, hip-distance apart, feet flexed and toes touching the floor so that you balance your body in a line like a plank (the top of a push-up).

Movement: Roll to the outer edge of your right foot, stacking your left foot on top of the right. Raise your left arm up toward the ceiling, palm forward with fingers extended and wrist aligned directly over your shoulder. Engage your abdominal muscles. Keeping your shoulders, hips, and feet in a straight line, balance on your right hand. Hold. Return to the starting position. Finish all reps, then repeat on your left side.

Tips and techniques:

- Keep your head and spine neutral, and directly align your shoulder over the hand on the floor.
- Focus on lifting your bottom hip.
- Keep your shoulders down and back.

Make it easier: Lying on your side, bend your top knee and place that foot on the floor in front of your other leg, toes pointing toward the wall in front of you. Keeping that foot on the floor, lift your hips.

Make it harder: From the full side plank, lift your top foot up toward the ceiling.

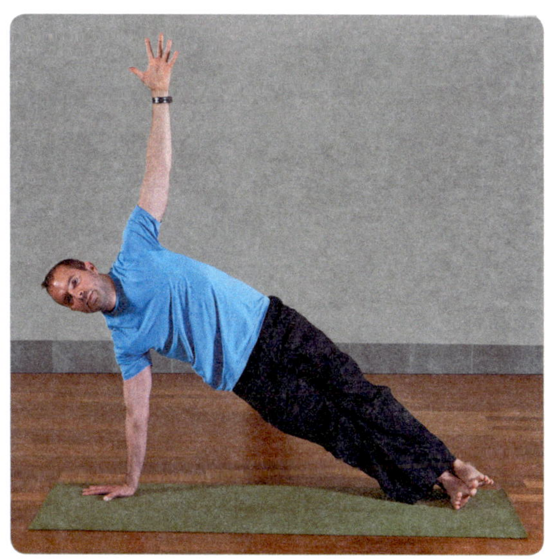

6 | Figure 4

Reps: 1 on each side
Sets: 1
Hold: 5 breaths

Starting position: Stand up straight, feet together, and weight evenly distributed on both feet. Relax your arms at your sides.

Movement: Standing on your right foot, bend your left knee and place your flexed left ankle above your right knee in a figure-4 position. To help you balance, press your left ankle firmly against your right leg and squeeze your right leg against your left ankle. Bring your arms to shoulder level, elbows slightly bent and palms inward. Now, extend your hips backward as if sitting down in a chair, while moving your arms forward to a wide V position. Tighten your abdominal muscles. Hold. Return to the starting position. Repeat the sequence standing on your left foot.

Tips and techniques:

- Exhale as you sink into the pose.
- Draw your shoulders down away from your ears.
- Breathe comfortably or practice yoga breathing.

Make it easier: Put your hand against a wall for support.

Make it harder: Hold for 10 breaths.

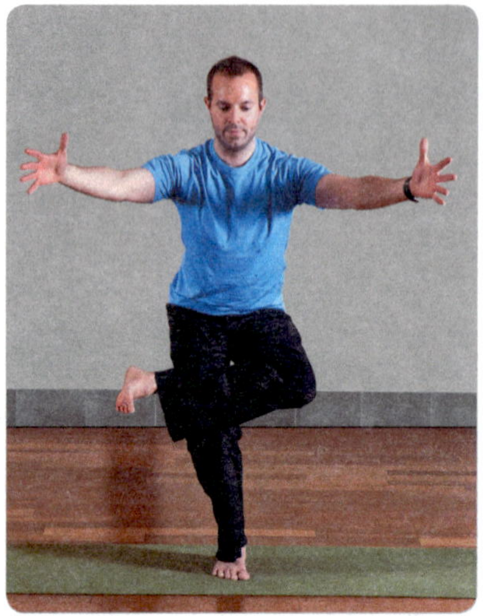

7 | Upward-facing dog

Reps: 2–4
Sets: 1
Hold: 5 breaths

Starting position: Lie facedown with your hands under your shoulders, elbows close to your sides. Extend your legs comfortably and press the tops of your feet against the floor.

Movement: Inhale, pushing with your hands and feet simultaneously to lift your torso and hips off the floor. Keep your chin parallel to the floor as you try to fully straighten your arms without locking your elbows. Hold. Return to the starting position.

Tips and techniques:

- Lift upward only to the point of mild tension, not pain.
- Do not lock your elbows when fully straightening your arms.
- Breathe comfortably or practice yoga breathing.

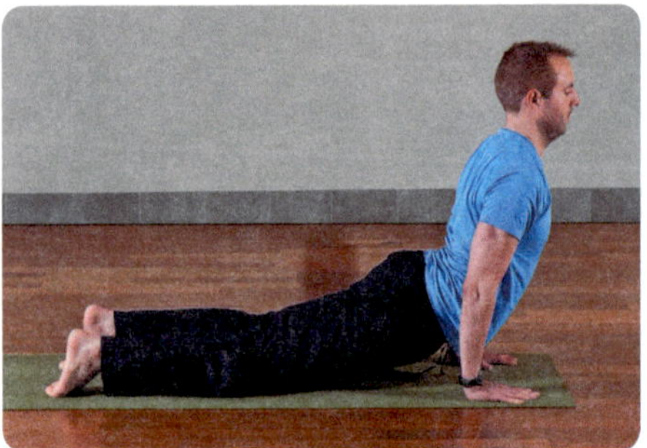

Make it easier: Do not lift upward as far, keeping your elbows bent.

Make it harder: Hold for 10 breaths.

8 | Downward-facing dog

Reps: 2–4
Sets: 1
Hold: 10 breaths

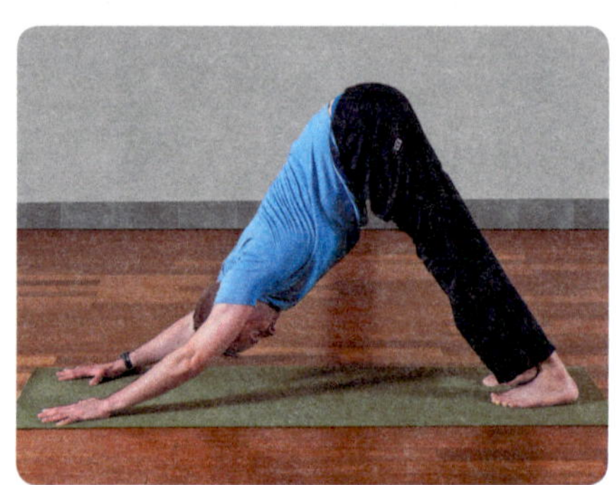

Starting position: Start on your hands and knees with your fingers extended and your toes tucked so the tops of your feet are off the floor.

Movement: Exhale as you lift your knees off the floor, straightening your legs without locking the knees until you are in an upside-down V. While maintaining a neutral neck and spine, align your ears with your biceps. Try to keep your weight evenly distributed between your hands and feet. Press your heels down toward the floor, if possible, while keeping your shoulders rolled back. Hold. Return to the starting position.

Tips and techniques:

- Keep your shoulders rolled back as you lengthen your spine.
- Tighten your abdominal muscles throughout.
- Breathe comfortably or practice yoga breathing.

Make it easier: Bend your knees slightly and let your heels come up off the floor.

Make it harder: Hold for 20 breaths.

▶ **You're not done yet.** See "Finish with stretches," page 47, for a set of seven stretches to end your routine. Stretching helps to prevent stiffness and preserve flexibility and range of motion.

Finish with stretches

Stretching is useful at any age and continues to be important into your 50s and beyond, even if you're less active than you once were. Stiffness can cause all kinds of problems. Your joints become less flexible over time. Stiff ankle and calf muscles may turn a trip into a tumble. Tight arm and side muscles may interfere with any task or sport involving reaching. Tight neck muscles may make it hard to look behind you, such as when you need to turn your head while backing up the car. Loss of flexibility undermines your balance, too, which can cause life-altering falls. Our stretches can help with all of these problems.

Perform stretches after your balance workout, when your muscles have been warmed up, to prevent injury. Aim to hold each stretch for a total of 60 seconds, doing as many repetitions as needed. For example, if you hold a stretch for 15 seconds, you would do four reps total.

Equipment: Cushioned mat, yoga strap for the hamstring stretch (page 48), sturdy chair for the calf stretch (page 49) and the standing quadriceps stretch (page 50).

1. Knees to chest

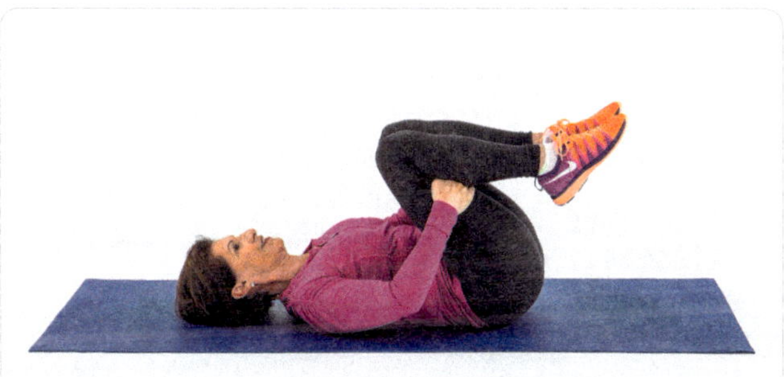

Primarily stretches the back

Reps: 2–6
Sets: 1
Hold: 10–30 seconds

Starting position: Lie on your back with your legs extended on the floor.

Movement: Relax your shoulders against the floor. Slowly bend your knees and pull them in toward your chest with your hands. Hold. Return to the starting position.

Tips and techniques:

- Stretch to the point of mild tension, not pain.
- When holding the stretch, remain as still as possible, without bouncing.
- Breathe comfortably.

2. Floor pretzel

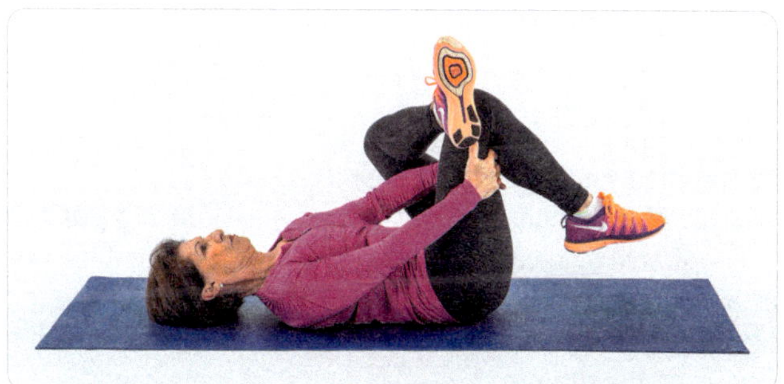

Primarily stretches the buttocks, hip, and outer thigh

Reps: 2–6
Sets: 1
Hold: 10–30 seconds

Starting position: Lie on your back with your right knee bent and foot on the floor. Rest your left ankle at the top of your right knee. Your left knee should point toward the wall. Grasp the back of your right thigh with both hands.

Movement: Keep your shoulders down and back, relaxing them against the floor. Slowly lift your right foot off the floor until you feel the stretch in your left hip and buttock. Hold. Return to the starting position. Repeat with your left knee bent and your right ankle resting on your left kneecap. This is one rep.

Tips and techniques:

- Stretch to the point of mild tension, not pain.
- If it's too hard to grasp your thigh with both hands, put a yoga strap or small towel around the back of the thigh and hold both ends.

3. Double knee torso rotation

Primarily stretches the back, chest, hip, and outer thigh

Reps: 2–6
Sets: 1
Hold: 10–30 seconds

Starting position: Lie on your back with your knees bent and feet together, flat on the floor. Put your arms out comfortably to each side at shoulder level, palms up.

Movement: Tighten your abdominal muscles and lift both knees toward your chest, then lower them together to the left side on the floor. Keeping your shoulders relaxed and pressed into the floor, look in the opposite direction. Feel the stretch across your chest and torso. Hold. Bring both knees back to center and return your right foot, then your left foot, to the floor. Repeat in the opposite direction. This is one rep.

Tips and techniques:

- Stretch to the point of mild tension, not pain.
- If necessary, put a rolled towel between your knees to make this stretch easier.
- Try to bring both knees up into a fetal position. Ideally, keep them together throughout the stretch.

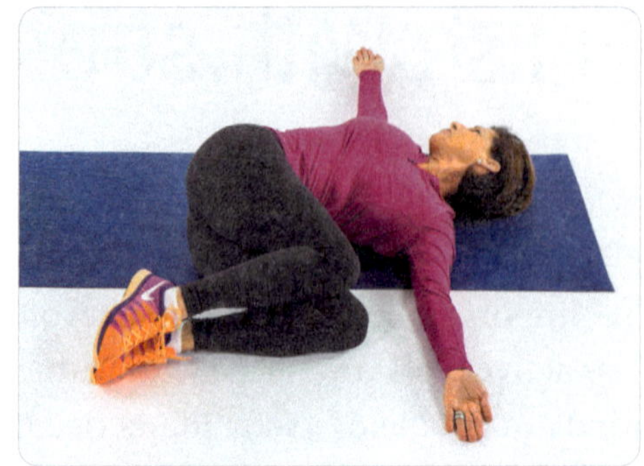

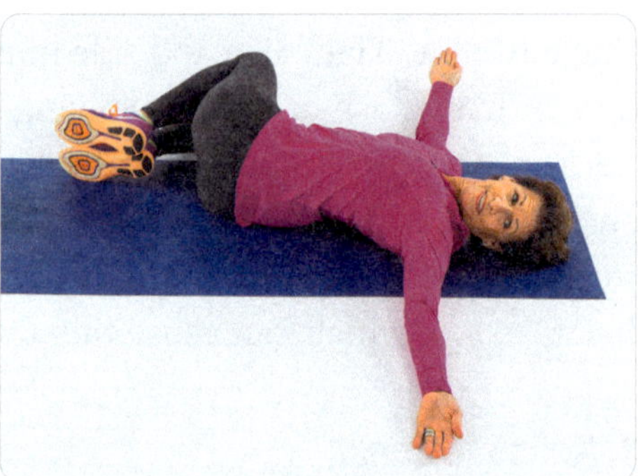

4. Hamstring stretch with strap

Primarily stretches the back of the thigh

The yoga strap used in this stretch helps you position yourself correctly even if your muscles are tight. It allows you to limit a stretch by keeping the strap long or, as your body becomes more flexible, to gently deepen a stretch by moving your grip up on the strap.

Reps: 2–6 on each side
Sets: 1
Hold: 10–30 seconds

Starting position: Lie on your back with your right leg extended on the floor. Bend your left knee to place the strap securely around your left foot. Hold the strap with both hands.

Movement: Flex the foot of your left leg and lift that heel toward the ceiling, straightening the leg as much as possible without locking the knee. As you do so, flex the foot of your extended right leg, pressing the thigh and calf down toward the floor. Gently pull on the strap to the point of muscle tightness. Hold. Return to the starting position. Finish all reps, then repeat with the legs reversed.

Tips and techniques:

- Stretch the leg that is raised toward the ceiling to the point of mild tension. You should not feel any pressure behind the knee.
- Place the strap in the middle of your foot to secure it safely.
- Breathe comfortably.

5. Kneeling hip flexor stretch

Primarily stretches the front of the hip

Reps: 2–6 on each side
Sets: 1
Hold: 10–30 seconds

Starting position: Kneel with your hands at your sides.

Movement: Put your right leg in front of you with the knee bent at a 90° angle and foot flat on the floor. Place your hands on your right thigh for support. Lean forward, pressing into the hip of your left leg while keeping your right foot on the floor. Hold. Return to the starting position. Finish all reps, then repeat on the other leg.

Tips and techniques:

- Stretch to the point of mild tension, not pain.
- Keep your head and spine neutral, your shoulders down and back, and your abdominal muscles tightened.
- Keep your spine neutral—don't arch your back.

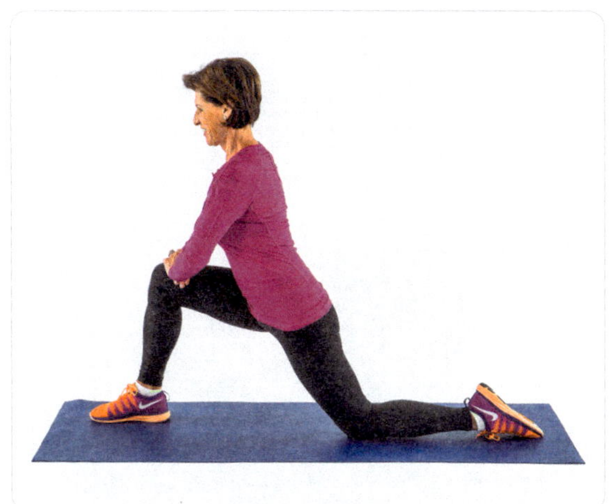

6. Calf stretch

Primarily stretches the calf, Achilles tendon, and ankle

Reps: 2–6
Sets: 1
Hold: 10–30 seconds

Starting position: Stand up straight. Hold the back of a chair or press your hands against a wall, arms extended at shoulder height.

Movement: Extend your right leg straight back and press the heel toward the floor. Allow your left knee to bend as you do so, while keeping that heel grounded on the floor. Hold. Return to the starting position, then repeat with your left leg. This is one rep.

Tips and techniques:

- Stretch to the point of mild tension, not pain.
- Hold a full-body lean from the ankle as you stretch.
- Maintain neutral posture with your shoulders down and back.

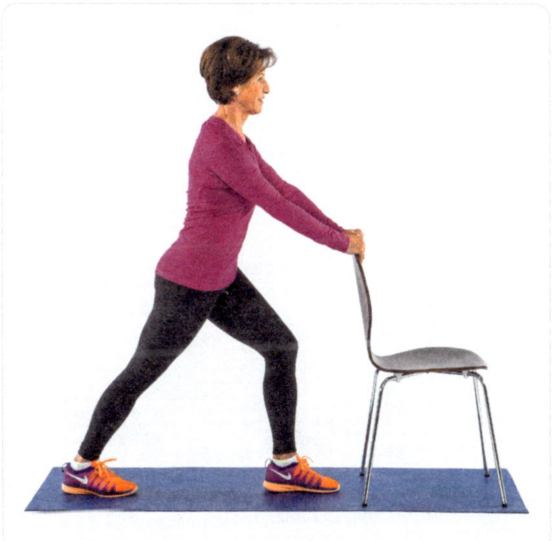

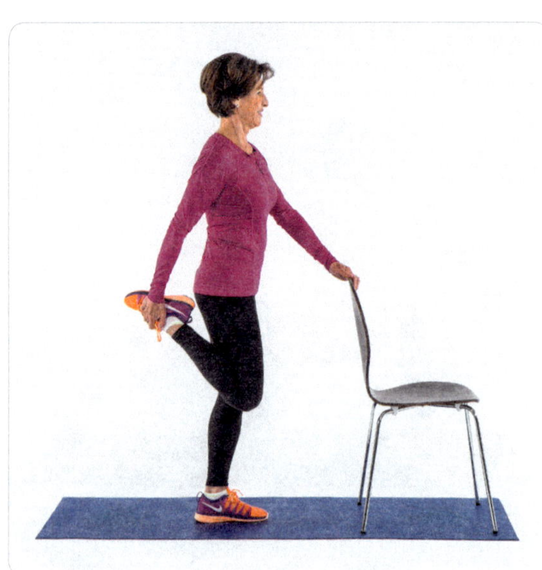

7. Standing quadriceps stretch

Primarily stretches the front of the thigh

Reps: 2–6
Sets: 1
Hold: 10–30 seconds

Starting position: Stand up straight, feet together, holding the back of a chair with both hands.

Movement: Bend your right knee and reach back with your right hand to grasp your foot, lifting it toward your right buttock. Keep your pelvis neutral. Hold. Slowly lower your foot to the floor. Switch position to repeat with your left leg. This is one rep.

Tips and techniques:

- Try to keep both knees together, with the bent knee pointing toward the floor.
- Stretch to the point of mild tension, not pain.
- If you have trouble grasping your foot, place a strap around it to assist with the stretch.

Note: Special thanks to the Equinox Fitness Club at 131 Dartmouth Street in Boston for the use of its facilities, and to the following Equinox personal trainers, instructors, and staff members for demonstrating the exercises depicted in this report: Josie Gardiner, Ian Lemieux, Joy Prouty, Cynthia Roth, and RaShaun Smith. The Yoga Balance Workout is reprinted from the Harvard Special Health Report *An Introduction to Yoga* and features Michele Stanten as the model. The stretches are excerpted from the Harvard Special Health Report *Stretching* and feature Josie Gardiner as the model.

Resources

Organizations

American Academy of Otolaryngology—Head and Neck Surgery
1650 Diagonal Road
Alexandria, VA 22314
703-836-4444
www.entnet.org

This is a national professional organization for specialists who treat problems of the ear, nose, and throat. Its website offers health information and a physician locator for the public.

American Academy of Physical Medicine and Rehabilitation
9700 W. Bryn Mawr Ave., Suite 200
Rosemont, IL 60018
847-737-6000
www.aapmr.org

This national professional organization for physiatrists—medical doctors trained in physical medicine and rehabilitation—provides information on conditions such as low back pain, neck pain, and osteoarthritis. The website includes a physician locator (go to "About physiatry" and click on "Find a PM&R physician").

American College of Sports Medicine
401 W. Michigan St.
Indianapolis, IN 46202
317-637-9200
www.acsm.org

ACSM is a nonprofit association that educates and certifies fitness professionals, such as personal trainers, and offers information to the public on various types of exercise. A referral service on the website locates ASCM-certified personal trainers (go to "Get & Stay Certified" and click on "Find a Pro").

American Council on Exercise
4933 Paramount Drive
San Diego, CA 92123
888-825-3636 (toll-free)
www.acefitness.org

ACE is a nonprofit organization that promotes fitness and offers educational materials for consumers and professionals. Its website offers a library of free exercise videos and a referral service to locate ACE-certified personal trainers and health coaches.

American Physical Therapy Association
3030 Potomac Ave., Suite 100
Alexandria, VA 22305
800-999-2782 (toll-free)
www.apta.org

This national professional organization fosters physical therapy education, research, and practice. Its companion website for the general public (www.choosept.com) provides educational articles and videos, plus a locator service.

Arthritis Foundation
1355 Peachtree St. NE, Suite 600
Atlanta, GA 30309
800-283-7800 (toll-free)
www.arthritis.org

This national nonprofit organization has local chapters in many states. The website offers educational materials on arthritis, pain control, standard medical treatments, and complementary therapies, along with podcasts hosted by people living with arthritis and Live Yes, an online support community. The foundation also offers Walk with Ease, a six-week walking program designed for people with arthritis.

Centers for Disease Control and Prevention
1600 Clifton Road
Atlanta, GA 30329
800-232-4636 (toll-free)
www.cdc.gov/steadi

This government agency created the STEADI (Stopping Elderly Accidents, Deaths & Injuries) initiative to reduce fall risk among older adults. The website provides a variety of information such as safety checklists, articles, and videos for the general public, along with resources for health care professionals.

National Institute on Aging
Building 31, Room 5C27
31 Center Drive, MSC 2292
Bethesda, MD 20892
800-222-2225 (toll-free)
www.nia.nih.gov/health/exercise-physical-activity

Part of the National Institutes of Health, the National Institute on Aging offers exercises, motivational tips, and free resources to help older adults get ready, start exercising, and keep going.

Vestibular Disorders Association
5018 NE 15th Ave.
Portland, OR 97211
800-837-8428 (800-VESTIBU; toll-free)
www.vestibular.org

This organization provides information on symptoms, diagnosis, and treatment of vestibular disorders. A provider directory can help you find a vestibular specialist in your area. You can also find support groups through the site.

Harvard Special Health Reports

The following Special Health Reports from Harvard Medical School may help improve your balance and reduce falls, either by boosting your strength and flexibility or by helping to correct ailments that impair balance. You can order by calling 877-649-9457 (toll-free) or going to www.health.harvard.edu.

The Aging Eye: Preventing and treating eye disease
Laura C. Fine, M.D., and Jeffrey S. Heier, M.D., Medical Editors
(Harvard Medical School, 2022)

Many eye disorders can contribute to fall risk. This report covers general vision problems, such as presbyopia, as well as specific ailments, including cataracts, glaucoma, age-related macular degeneration, and diabetic retinopathy.

Better Bladder and Bowel Control: Practical strategies for managing incontinence
May M. Wakamatsu, M.D.; Elise J.B. De, M.D.; and Liliana Bordeianou, M.D., Medical Editors
(Harvard Medical School, 2021)

Though treating incontinence will not improve your balance directly, it can reduce fall risk, since many people fall when rushing to the bathroom. This report covers multiple solutions for both urinary and fecal incontinence.

Coping with Hearing Loss: A guide to prevention and treatment
David Murray Vernick, M.D., and Ann Gentili-Stockwell, M.A., Medical Editors
(Harvard Medical School, 2019)

Inner-ear issues can contribute to balance problems. This report discusses different types of hearing loss and possible solutions. It includes an extensive section on the many options in hearing aids.

Core Exercises: 6 workouts to tighten your abs, strengthen your back, and improve balance
Lauren E. Elson, M.D., Medical Editor, with Michele Stanten, Fitness Consultant
(Harvard Medical School, 2020)

Strong core muscles underlie almost everything you do, from walking to playing sports. These six workouts help build core strength, which helps you to be more stable whether you're standing still or moving.

Gentle Core Exercises: Start toning your abs, building your back muscles, and reclaiming core fitness today
Lauren E. Elson, M.D., Medical Editor, with Michele Stanten, Fitness Consultant
(Harvard Medical School, 2020)

This special program of gentle core exercises lets you get started in a safe, easy way, if you've had an injury, you've been unwell, you're afraid you'll hurt yourself, or you're concerned that you might make an existing injury worse.

Intermediate Yoga: Deepen your practice to find more strength, flexibility, energy, and happiness
Darshan Mehta, M.D., M.P.H., Medical Editor, and Laura Malloy, L.I.C.S.W.
(Harvard Medical School, 2021)

Building on basic yoga poses and breathing techniques, this report offers six targeted routines, including one designed to improve balance, for those who already have experience with yoga. If you're a beginner, see *An Introduction to Yoga*, above right.

An Introduction to Tai Chi: A gentle exercise program for mental and physical well-being
Peter M. Wayne, Ph.D., Medical Editor
(Harvard Medical School, 2022)

Research shows that tai chi reduces both the risk of falling and the fear of falling. This basic program helps improve balance, posture, body awareness, coordination, and strength.

An Introduction to Yoga: Improve your strength, balance, flexibility, and well-being
Sat Bir Singh Khalsa, Ph.D., and Lauren E. Elson, M.D., Medical Editors (Harvard Medical School, 2020)

With so many types of yoga, where do you begin? This report provides a safe, simple program, including sitting, standing, and floor exercises that can help with balance and flexibility. The Yoga Balance Workout (page 32) is drawn from this report.

The Joint Pain Relief Workout: Healing exercises for your shoulders, hips, knees, and ankles
Lauren E. Elson, M.D., Medical Editor, with Michele Stanten, Fitness Consultant
(Harvard Medical School, 2021)

Pain can make you more susceptible to falling if it distracts you and impairs nerve and muscle responses. But the right set of exercises can help control ankle, knee, hip, or shoulder pain and may help you postpone or avoid surgery on a problem joint.

Living Well with Osteoarthritis: A guide to relieving the pain and caring for your joints
Robert H. Shmerling, M.D., Medical Editor
(Harvard Medical School, 2019)

Arthritis pain can make you unsteady on your feet when it causes you to alter your gait. This report discusses many ways of managing arthritis pain, from physical therapy to surgery. A special section covers self-care strategies for coping with arthritis.

Strength and Power Training for All Ages: 4 complete workouts to tone up, slim down, and get fit
Elizabeth Pegg Frates, M.D., Medical Editor, with Michele Stanten, Fitness Consultant
(Harvard Medical School, 2021)

Weak muscles make it harder to stay active and can impair balance and coordination. These four complete workouts allow you to progress from easy to hard strength and power exercises. The report includes a section on plyometrics (jump training).

Strength and Power Training for Older Adults: Two complete workouts to start rebuilding your muscles
Elizabeth Pegg Frates, M.D., Medical Editor, with Michele Stanten, Fitness Consultant
(Harvard Medical School, 2019)

This report provides a basic program designed specifically to help older adults build strength as well as power—the boost that adds speed to strength to help you walk faster or react more quickly, so that a trip doesn't become a fall.

Stretching: 35 stretches to improve flexibility and reduce pain
Lauren E. Elson, M.D., Medical Editor, with Michele Stanten, Fitness Consultant
(Harvard Medical School, 2017)

Stretches can help relieve back pain, stiff necks, and sore knees when tight muscles are to blame. As you age, they can also help keep you active and flexible. The stretches provided in Better Balance (see "Finish with stretches," page 47) are examples of what you will find in the *Stretching* Special Health Report.